D0221805

THOMSON DELMAR LEARNING'S
CASE STUDY SERIES

Maternity

&

Women's Health

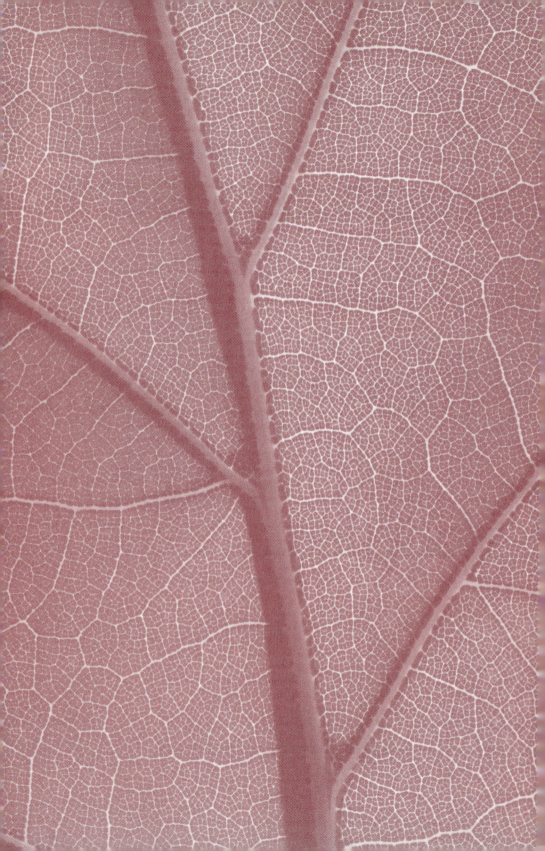

Contents

Reviewers

Denise G. Link, NPC, DNSc
Women's Health Care Nurse Practitioner
Clinical Associate Professor
Arizona State University
Tempe, Arizona

Tamella Livengood, APRN, BC, MSN, FNP
Nursing Faculty, Northwestern Michigan College
Traverse City, Michigan

Vicki Nees, RNC, MSN, APRN-BC
Associate Professor
Ivy Tech State College
Lafayette, Indiana

Patricia Posey-Goodwin, MSN, RN, EdD (c)
Assistant Professor
University of West Florida
Pensacola, Florida

Series Preface

Thomson Delmar Learning's Case Studies Series was created to encourage nurses to bridge the gap between content knowledge and clinical application. The products within the series represent the most innovative and comprehensive approach to nursing case studies ever developed. Each title has been authored by experienced nurse educators and clinicians who understand the complexity of nursing practice as well as the challenges of teaching and learning. All of the cases are based on real-life clinical scenarios and demand thought and "action" from the nurse. Each case brings the user into the clinical setting and invites the reader to utilize the nursing process while considering all of the variables that influence the client's condition and the care to be provided. Each case also represents a unique set of variables to offer a breadth of learning experiences and to capture the reality of nursing practice. To gauge the progression of a user's knowledge and critical thinking ability, the cases have been categorized by difficulty level. Every section begins with basic cases and proceeds to more advanced scenarios, thereby presenting opportunities for learning and practice for both students and professionals.

All of the cases have been reviewed by experts to ensure that as many variables as possible are represented in a truly realistic manner and that each case reflects consistency with realities of modern nursing practice.

How to Use This Book

Every case begins with a table of variables that are encountered in practice and that must be understood by the nurse in order to provide appropriate care to the client. Categories of variables include age, setting, ethnicity, cultural considerations, pre-existing conditions, co-existing conditions, communication considerations, disability considerations, socioeconomic considerations, spiritual considerations, pharmacological considerations, psychosocial considerations, legal considerations, ethical considerations, alternative therapy, prioritization considerations, and delegation considerations. If a case involves a variable that is considered to have a significant impact on care, the specific variable is included in the table. This allows the user an "at a glance" view of the issues that will need to be considered to provide care to the client in the scenario. The table of variables is followed by a presentation of the case, including the history of the client, current condition, clinical setting, and professionals involved. A series of questions follows each case that ask the user to consider how to handle the issues presented within the scenario. Suggested answers and rationales are provided for remediation and discussion.

Organization

The cases are grouped into parts based on topics. Within each part, cases are organized by difficulty level from easy, to moderate, to difficult. The classifications are somewhat subjective, but they are based upon a developed standard. In general, difficulty level has been determined by the number of variables that impact the case and the complexity of the client's condition. Colored tabs are used to allow the user to distinguish the difficulty levels more easily. A comprehensive table of variables is also provided for reference to allow the user to quickly select cases containing a particular variable of care.

Praise for Thomson Delmar Learning's Case Study Series

I would recommend this book to my undergraduate students. This would be a required book for graduate students in nursing education, women's health, or maternal–child programs.

PATRICIA POSEY-GOODWIN, MSN, RN, EdD (c)
Assistant Professor
University of West Florida

This text does an excellent job of reflecting the complexity of nursing practice.

VICKI NEES, RNC, MSN, APRN-BC
Associate Professor
Ivy Tech State College

. . . [T]he case studies are very comprehensive and allow the undergraduate student an opportunity to apply knowledge gained in the classroom to a potentially real clinical situation.

TAMELLA LIVENGOOD, APRN, BC, MSN, FNP
Nursing Faculty
Northwestern Michigan College

I commend the effort to include the impact of illness on the growth and development of the child, on the family's cohesiveness, and on the subsequent health problems that will affect the child in years to come. Inclusion of questions that focus on the nurse's perceptions, biases, and beliefs are extremely important when training nurses to provide comprehensive care . . . Often one system illness will affect another health system, and this has been demonstrated numerous times [in this text].

DIANA JACOBSON
MS, RN, CPNP
Faculty Associate
Arizona State University College of Nursing

These cases and how you have approached them definitely stimulate the students to use critical-thinking skills. I thought the questions asked really pushed the students to think deeply and thoroughly.

JOANNE SOLCHANY, PhD, ARNP, RN, CS
Assistant Professor, Family & Child Nursing
University of Washington

The use of case studies is pedagogically sound and very appealing to students and instructors. I think that some instructors avoid them because of the challenge of case development. You have provided the material for them.

NANCY L. OLDENBURG, RN, MS, CPNP
Clinical Instructor
Northern Illinois University

[The author] has done an excellent job of assisting students to engage in critical thinking. I am very impressed with the cases, questions, and content. I rarely ask that students buy more than one pediatrics book . . . but, in this instance, I can't wait until this book is published.

DEBORAH J. PERSELL, MSN, RN, CPNP
Assistant Professor
Arkansas State University

This is a groundbreaking book that . . . will be appropriate for undergraduate pediatric courses as well as a variety of graduate programs . . . One of the most impressive features is the variety of cases that cover situations from primary care through critical care and rehabilitation. The cases are presented to develop and assess critical-thinking skills . . . All cases are framed within a comprehensive presentation of physical findings, stimulating critical thinking about pathophysiology, developmental considerations, and family systems. This book should be a required text for all undergraduate and graduate nursing programs and should be well-received by faculty.

JANE H. BARNSTEINER, PhD, RN, FAAN
Professor of Pediatric Nursing
University of Pennsylvania School of Nursing

Preface

Case Studies Series: Maternity and Women's Health has been developed to provide the student with an opportunity to experience a wide range of clinical encounters in women's health. The case format provides the opportunity to move from theory to application. It provides users with a transitional tool to guide students into practice. The case studies format gives users the opportunity to utilize the nursing process in order to make decisions based on multiple variables. The clients, although fictitious, are presented as believable characters in multicultural, realistic scenarios, removing as much as possible the situations from isolated text theory and asking students to relate to the persons as individuals. It is the intention that adding this realism will guide the user into focusing on the whole person and their responses to health changes, not merely on the physical processes.

Empowerment of women and their families is maintained as an essential core in this process. Currently, providers of maternity care are faced with the high risk associated with malpractice suits and financial constraints as a result of reduced reimbursement and increased insurance cost. This often results in pressure to provide "medical-legal" care. The nurse, practicing the advocacy role, provides the balance that keeps care client-centered. Often this is difficult because nursing itself struggles with downsizing and short staffing. A concerted effort has been made to apply current evidence-based science and to guide the user into the exploration of both short-term and long-term effects of routine non-evidence-based interventions. Nurses who have a confident grasp of evidence-based care are better prepared to intervene for their client's well-being. Users are encouraged to stay current on newer evidence-based studies as they are released and revisit cases to apply this knowledge as it becomes available.

Organization

Cases are grouped according to phases in the childbearing cycle. Prenatal cases are presented initially, followed by intrapartum, newborn, and then postpartum. These are followed by cases in non-maternity-related women's health. The cases are fictitious; however, they are based on actual problems and/or situations the nurse will encounter throughout a career in women's health. Any resemblance to actual cases or individuals is coincidental.

To assist in selecting cases, each case is preceded by a blueprint listing the specific variables being presented in the case. For example, the following information is listed when it is pertinent for that case: Client age, setting, ethnicity, significant history factors, pre-existing conditions, co-existing conditions, communication problems, disabilities, socioeconomic factors, spiritual or religious factors, prioritization concerns, legal and ethical concerns, need for delegation, pharmacologic agents, and alternative therapies referred to in the case. The level of difficulty is identified at the start of the case, and a brief overview is provided.

The case is then presented starting with a client profile to provide background followed by the scenario. Each scenario is followed by a series of questions. Answers and rationales follow each question at the end of the case study.

In addition to cases that focus on the client disease and responses to disease, the scenarios are presented in multicultural settings, which present real ethical and moral dilemmas that nurses are facing in the workplace and the community. In the more advanced cases the user is asked to utilize critical thinking, apply the nursing process, and use professional judgment to critique the care provided. Students are asked to review routine interventions in light of evidence-based studies for both evidence efficacy and the impact of these interventions on safety and the quality of the care provided.

Several cases present social problems reflecting flaws in the current provider networks. The user is presented with clients who have "fallen through the cracks" in the system and is asked to explore ways that the professional nurse can become proactive to bring about social change for better delivery of care.

Acknowledgments

My sincere thanks to Maria D'Angelico, Developmental Editor, and the entire editorial staff at Thomson Delmar Learning for guidance in writing this text and making it a reality. A special thank you to Justine Clegg for reviewing the case on grieving. Justine's years of experience as both a certified professional midwife and mental health counselor were valuable to completing this case. Thank you to Heather Gordon for reviewing and contributing to several of the well woman and neonatal cases. I would also like to thank the reviewers for their time and valuable input.

Dedication

This book is dedicated to my husband, John, our children, and their families for their continued support and encouragement through this very long process. A special dedication of this book goes to Janice Heller, CPM and my friend, and to the many dedicated midwives and nurses who still believe in normal birth and who have spent a lifetime empowering women who seek holistic family-centered care and out-of-hospital birth. As long as you are out there, normal birth will be safe.

About the Author

Diann S. Gregory received her BSN at Madonna University in 1969. Diann's grandmother Robertson guided her in the direction of nursing and her mother's courage and dad's challenge made it possible to go to college. She received her MSEd in adult education from Florida International University, and her Nurse Midwifery Certificate in 1998 from the Frontier School of Nursing and Midwifery (CNEP program). Diann started her nursing career in the Army Nurse Corps as an operating room nurse in Viet Nam where she received a bronze star for her work in surgery and volunteer work at the local orphanage.

She has spent over 36 years working as staff nurse, patient educator, clinical specialist, and nursing faculty at the associate and bachelor's level and has been a preceptor at the masters level in the field of Women's Health. For the past 12 years she has taught direct entry midwifery at Miami Dade College. Diann earned her RNC in 1986 from the NAACOG Certification Corp. and is a Lamaze certified instructor. Over the past nine years on three different occasions, Diann has been honored by her peers to receive the highest honor awarded to Miami Dade College professors, the three-year Endowed Teaching Chair. She has also twice been awarded the NISOD award for teaching excellence from the University of Texas at Austin. Recently she was recognized as a finalist in The Thomas Ehrlich Faculty Award for Service-Learning, an annual national award that recognizes leaders in community service learning.

Her contributions to education include authoring several video teaching tapes in the series "ABC of Nursing" produced at Miami Dade College, one of which, "Intrapartum Care," received first place from the National League for Nursing in 1993. Through grants, she created and developed interactive virtual practices for teaching antepartum to midwifery students. This program has been presented at several national conferences. She was instrumental in obtaining grants to develop a program to train doulas and has her own consulting business working with hospitals in the areas of quality assurance and risk management. For over 20 years Diann has worked as a legal consultant to legal firms in three counties. She is currently a full time professor in the nursing and midwifery programs at Miami Dade College.

Diann married her combat buddy from Viet Nam. John was a medical evacuation DUSTOFF helicopter pilot, and is her lifetime hero. They dated in combat boots and he won her heart as he would daily put the lives of the soldiers in the field above his own as he headed into active combat zones to bring them into her hospital. They have been married for 34 years and have four children.

Diann has been blessed to be doula for their daughter Diann and husband, Dan, during their three difficult high-risk deliveries. On the request of her daughter-in-law, two years ago she flew to Korea where their son John, an Army officer, was stationed. There she was honored to be the midwife to her daughter-in-law, Yali, and guided her through the birth of a granddaughter. John and Yali's five-year-old daughter provided assistance. John and Diann's youngest daughter, Josie, and husband, Sam, look forward to her support in the near future as they plan their family. John and Diann's youngest, Tony, has proudly become a Florida Gator this year as he enters his junior year at the University of Florida. Family has filled Diann's life with love that she has been able to bring to each of her clients and students over many years.

Diann may be reached at Miami Dade College, Medical Center Campus, 950 NW 20th Street, Miami, Florida 33127. She may also be contacted by e-mail at dgregory@mdc.edu or by phone at (305) 237-4460.

Comprehensive Table of Variables

Part 1: Prenatal Case Studies

CASE STUDY	AGE	SETTING	CULTURAL CONSIDERATIONS	ETHNICITY	PRE-EXISTING CONDITION	CO-EXISTING CONDITION/CURRENT PROBLEM	COMMUNICATIONS	DISABILITY	SOCIOECONOMIC STATUS	SPIRITUAL/RELIGIOUS	PSYCHOSOCIAL	LEGAL	ETHICAL	PRIORITIZATION	DELEGATION	PHARMACOLOGIC	ALTERNATIVE THERAPY	SIGNIFICANT HISTORY
1	26	Public health clinic	Caribbean culture; Hispanic traditions	Hispanic American		x			x									x
2	28	Midwifery private practice	Vietnamese/Buddhist culture	Asian American						x						x		x
3	37	Midwifery prenatal clinic	Orthodox Jewish culture	Jewish American	x	x				x	x							x
4	26	Private OB setting	Muslim tradition	Middle Eastern	x					x								x
5	16	High school health clinic	Black American impoverished mores	Black American	x	x			x		x	x						x
6	22	Prenatal clinic	Dominican Republican traditions	Black/Caribbean Islander		x			x		x					x		x
7	32	Client's home	Hispanic American culture	Hispanic American second-generation	x	x				x						x		x
8	28	Public health clinic	Mexican culture; immigrant community	Hispanic	x											x	x	

Part 2: Intrapartum Case Studies

CASE STUDY	AGE	SETTING	CULTURAL CONSIDERATIONS	ETHNICITY	PRE-EXISTING CONDITION	CO-EXISTING CONDITION/CURRENT PROBLEM	COMMUNICATIONS	DISABILITY	SOCIOECONOMIC STATUS	SPIRITUAL/RELIGIOUS	PSYCHOSOCIAL	LEGAL	ETHICAL	PRIORITIZATION	DELEGATION	PHARMACOLOGIC	ALTERNATIVE THERAPY	SIGNIFICANT HISTORY
1	29	Birth center	Second-generation Cuban immigrant traditions	Hispanic American	x	x					x							x

xix

Abbreviations Commonly Used in Maternity and Women's Health Nursing

ABR . . . . auditory brainstem response

AFI. . . . . amniotic fluid index

AFP. . . . . alpha fetoprotein

AGCUS . . . . atypical glandular cells of undetermined significance

AMA . . . . advanced maternal age

AROM . . . . artificial rupture of membranes

ASCUS. . . . . . . atypical squamous cells of undetermined significance

BMI . . . . body mass index

BMR . . . . basal metabolic rate

BP. . . . . blood pressure

BPD . . . . bronchopulmonary dysplasia

BPP . . . . biophysical profile

BV . . . . bacterial vaginosis

CNM . . . . certified nurse midwife

CVAT . . . . costovertebral angle tenderness

CVS . . . . chorionic villus sampling

CPD. . . . . cephalopelvic disproportion

CPM . . . certified professional midwife

DIC . . . . disseminated intravascular coagulopathy

DVT . . . . deep vein thrombosis

EBL . . . . estimated blood loss

EFW. . . . . estimated fetal weight

EOAD . . . . evoked otoacoustic emission test

FH . . . . fundal height

FHT. . . . . fetal heart tone

FM. . . . . fetal movement

fob . . . . father of the baby

FSE . . . . fetal scalp electrode

FSH. . . . . follicle-stimulating hormone

FTP . . . . failure to progress

GBS . . . . group B streptococcus

hCG. . human chorionic gonadotropin

H&H . . . . hematocrit and hemoglobin

H&P . . . . history and physical

HA . . . . headache

HELLP. . . . hemolysis elevated liver enzymes and low platclets

HRT . . hormone replacement therapy

HSIL . . . . high grade squamous intraepithelial lesions

I&O . . . . intake and output

IDM . . . . infant of diabetic mother

IUGR . . . . intrauterine growth retardation

IUP . . . . intrauterine pregnancy

IUPC . . intrauterine pressure catheter

KVO . . . . keep vein open

LLQ . . . . left lower quadrant

LNMP . . last normal menstrual period

LOA . . . . left occiput anterior

LSB . . . . lower sternal border

LSIL . low-grade squamous intraepithelial lesions

LTV . . . . long-term variablility

MAS. . meconium aspiration syndrome

MgSO$_4$ . . magnesium sulfate (JCAHO recommends that use of this abbreviation be discontinued because of its potential for being confused with the abbreviation for morphine sulfate)

MMS . . . . . multiple marker screening

NEC. . . . . . . necrotizing enterocolitis

NSVD. . . . . normal spontaneous vaginal delivery

OCP . . . . oral contraceptive pills

ONTD . . . . . open neural tube defects

PDA. . . . . patent ductus arteriosis

PID . . . . . . pelvic inflammatory disease

PMI . . . . point of maximal impulse

PPV . . . . . positive pressure ventilation

PPW . . . . pre-pregnancy weight

PPROM . . . . preterm premature rupture of membranes

PROM . . . . premature rupture of membranes

PTL . . . . preterm labor

RDS . . . . respiratory distress syndrome

R/O. . . . . rule out

r/t. . . . . related to

S < D . . . . size less than dates

SIDS . . sudden infant death syndrome

SIL . . squamous intraepithelial lesions

SROM. . . . . spontaneous rupture of membranes

STI . . . . sexually transmitted infection (also known as STD—sexually transmitted disease)

T. . . . . temperature

TENS . . . . transcutaneous electrical nerve stimulator

Toc . . . . test of cure

TOP. . . . . . . termination of pregnancy

TPN . . . . total parenteral nutrition

TTN . . . . transient tachypnea of the newborn

URQ. . . . . upper right quadrant

UTI . . . . urinary tract infection

VBAC . . . . vaginal birth after cesarean

VE . . . . vaginal exam

VS . . . . vital signs

wga . . . . weeks gestational age

wnl . . . . within normal limits

THOMSON DELMAR LEARNING'S
CASE STUDY SERIES

Maternity

&

Women's Health

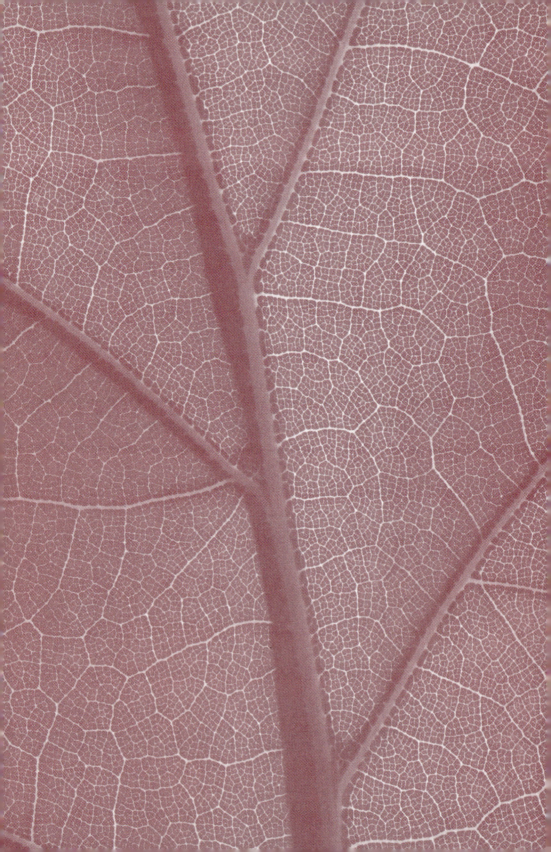

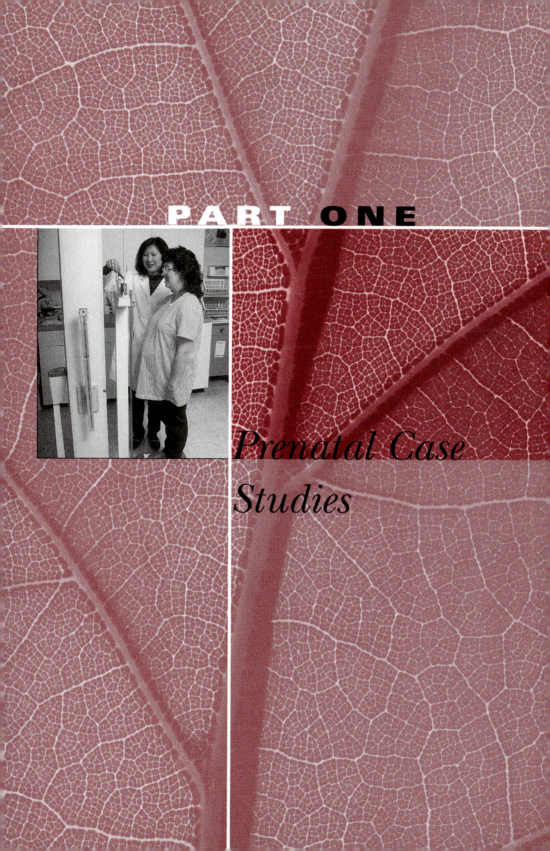

PART ONE

Prenatal Case Studies

Paola

AGE

26

SETTING

- Public health clinic

CULTURAL CONSIDERATIONS

- Caribbean culture; Hispanic traditions

ETHNICITY

- Hispanic American

PRE-EXISTING CONDITION

CO-EXISTING CONDITION/CURRENT PROBLEM

- Closely spaced pregnancies; lead exposure; S < D; pica; late entry to care; headaches

COMMUNICATIONS

DISABILITY

SOCIOECONOMIC STATUS

- Poverty

SPIRITUAL/RELIGIOUS

PSYCHOSOCIAL

LEGAL

ETHICAL

PRIORITIZATION

DELEGATION

PHARMACOLOGIC

ALTERNATIVE THERAPY

SIGNIFICANT HISTORY

- History of stillbirth; multigravida

PRENATAL, second trimester

Level of difficulty: Easy

Overview: This case requires that the student consider the environmental factors and their effects on the health of the mother, fetus, and three-year-old child.

Client Profile

Paola is a 26-year-old, G3P1101. She, her husband, and their three-year-old moved to the Florida Keys two years ago from Santa Domingo. Last year she had a stillbirth at 30 wga. The cause of the stillbirth was not determined. She did not have prenatal care and never went back to the clinic for postpartum follow-up.

Case Study

Paola is now 19 wga and is attending the prenatal clinic for an initial prenatal visit. She is five feet two inches tall, and her current weight is 126 pounds, which is four pounds over her pre-pregnancy weight (PPW). She is concerned about this baby because of her loss last year. The following data was obtained at this visit:

- S < D
- BP 110/60
- +FM
- FHT LLQ 150–160s
- Complains of intermittent headaches with no vision changes

The nurse also notes that the three-year-old is hyperactive and very small for her age. She engages Paola in a conversation and discovers that they live in a small apartment over a convenience store attached to a gas station. The family gets the apartment rent-free because her husband watches the station during the night. In the daytime he is a mechanic there. Paola also does extra laundry (workers' uniforms and rags from the garage) in her home to help supplement the income.

Questions

1. Identify at least two possible reasons why Paola did not receive prenatal care or go for follow-up care after her last pregnancy, and why she is starting prenatal care so late with this pregnancy.

2. Is there a possible connection between the three-year-old daughter's development and Paola's pregnancy history?

3. What lab work should the nurse anticipate (other than the routine initial lab work)?

4. Identify at least five possible sources of lead exposure for Paola and her family.

5. Paola's lead level at 19 wga was high. It was rechecked at 28 wga and had fallen.

At 36 wga it had again risen. Why, and what is the significance of this pattern?

6. What are the health risks for Paola from lead exposure?

7. Is lead a teratogen?

8. What are the consequences of high lead levels for the newborn/child?

9. What interventions can the nurse offer Paola during the pregnancy to reduce her exposure and consequences of the lead for herself, her three-year-old, and the fetus?

10. Paola delivers a 4½-pound baby at 37 weeks. She would like to breastfeed. What should the nurse advise?

Questions and Suggested Answers

1. Identify at least two possible reasons why Paola did not receive prenatal care or go for follow-up care after her last pregnancy, and why she is starting prenatal care so late with this pregnancy. Hispanic women tend to be present oriented. She may not have seen the need for prenatal care or realized how it could influence the outcome of her pregnancy. Another culturally related characteristic in Hispanic women is the tendency to accept outcomes as fate. "It doesn't matter what I do, the outcome is already predetermined" (Simpson, 2001). A second reason is poverty, which can interfere with the ability to travel to care, ability to pay for care, and ability to take off work to go for care.

2. Is there a possible connection between the three-year-old daughter's development and Paola's pregnancy history? They both could be exhibiting effects of lead toxicity.

3. What lab work should the nurse anticipate (other than the routine initial lab work)? Other lab work that needs to be done includes serum lead levels and free protoporphyrin levels.

4. Identify at least five possible sources of lead exposure for Paola and her family. Paola could have lead storage in her system from leaded gasoline used in Santo Domingo. Other sources are the ground around the gas station. This would be even worse if she has pica, a condition that may cause her to eat the dirt. The air around the gas station from the car exhaust may also contribute to the lead exposure. Finally, one of the worst sources of lead is the batteries stored at the garage/gas station. The lead in the ground may be taken into vegetables if she has a garden. The water may be contaminated near the station, and they may be using water from a shallow well. This is no longer common, but it is a possibility.

5. Paola's lead level at 19 wga was high. It was rechecked at 28 wga and had fallen. At 36 wga it had again risen. Why, and what is the significance of this pattern? The high levels initially could be a result of increased maternal absorption in pregnancy. When she was checked at 28 weeks, her levels may have fallen due to the fetus taking the lead. In later pregnancy, the levels tend to rise again, possibly due to maternal bone demineralization (Hackley, 2003).

6. What are the health risks for Paola from lead exposure? She is at a higher risk for pre-eclampsia, anemia, and decreased cognitive levels with aging if bone demineralization occurs at menopause and increased lead is released into her circulation.

7. Is lead a teratogen? Lead has not been proven to be a teratogen in itself; however, it is a neurotoxin and does show an association with minor deformities.

8. What are the consequences of high lead levels for the newborn/child? Cognitive damage may occur decreasing the child's ability to perform on verbal and nonverbal reasoning, math, and short-term memory tests. Lower IQ and antisocial behavior have also been identified. Low birth weight is also common. When the lead exposure is corrected during the postnatal period, the infants will usually catch up on their weight.

9. What interventions can the nurse offer Paola during the pregnancy to reduce her exposure and consequences of the lead for herself, her three-year-old, and the fetus? Dietary guidance, including:

- Avoid fasting.
- Increase vitamin C intake.
- Increase calcium intake.
- Increase iron intake and, if anemic, take supplements.
- Reduce exposure—in her case she could have her husband do his own laundry and she should not be doing the garage workers' laundry or rags from the garage.
- Use special water filters on water taps.
- If she smokes, encourage her to stop since this increases lead absorption.
- Avoid eating dirt (pica—if that had been a problem).
- Do not use improperly fired ceramicware when cooking or storing foods since these often contain lead that is easily released into the food.
- Move, if that is feasible. If not, keep windows closed on the sides of the apartment that have the most exposure to fumes from the garage and gas station.
- The child should be referred to a pediatric specialist who has experience in lead poisoning.

10. Paola delivers a 4½-pound baby at 37 weeks. She would like to breastfeed. What should the nurse advise? This will depend on her lead levels. If they are less than 35 mcg/dl, she should be encouraged to breastfeed. Breast milk is so superior to formula that her levels must be very high before a recommendation to bottle-feed is given. Another point is that formula also contains lead, and switching to formula may not reduce the baby's exposure at all. If she is mixing powdered formula and using well water, the water may also contain lead. If she is breastfeeding, she needs to take calcium supplements since they will prevent bone demineralization. Adequate iron and vitamin C also help reduce the amount of lead transferred during breastfeeding.

References

Hackley, B., & Katz-Jacobson, A. (2003). Lead poisoning in pregnancy: a case study with implications for midwives. *Journal of Midwifery and Woman's Health, 48*(1), 30–38.

Simpson, K. R, & Creehan, P. A. (2001). *AWHONN perinatal nursing* (2nd ed.). Philadelphia: Lippincott, Williams & Wilkins.

Allyson

AGE

28

SETTING

- Midwifery private practice

CULTURAL CONSIDERATIONS

- Vietnamese/Buddhist culture

ETHNICITY

- Asian American

PRE-EXISTING CONDITION

CO-EXISTING CONDITION/CURRENT PROBLEM

COMMUNICATIONS

DISABILITY

SOCIOECONOMIC STATUS

SPIRITUAL/RELIGIOUS

- Buddhist

PSYCHOSOCIAL

LEGAL

ETHICAL

PRIORITIZATION

DELEGATION

PHARMACOLOGIC

- Vitamin B_6; promethazine (Phenergan); prochlorperazine (Compazine)

ALTERNATIVE THERAPY

SIGNIFICANT HISTORY

- Primigravida; attempted pregnancy for three years

PRENATAL, first trimester

Level of difficulty: Moderate

Overview: This case asks the students to determine the due date and the number of weeks gestation the pregnancy is. It requires that the student be able to identify some of the common discomforts and distinguish them from warning signs in early pregnancy. Specifically, students must also be able to assess early pregnancy spotting and identify signs and symptoms associated with ectopic pregnancy.

Client Profile

Allyson is a 28-year-old, G1P0, married Vietnamese American. She and her husband have been trying to achieve pregnancy for three years. Allyson works as a bank teller; her husband is a bank manager. They have lots of family support since both families live within 30 minutes of them. They are constantly reminded that their parents want grandchildren. Allyson is five feet two inches, and her current weight is 118 pounds. She states, "I did a home pregnancy test yesterday and it was positive! My last menstrual period was exactly six weeks ago. I can't believe I am pregnant. I feel great!" Her physical exam (PE) is within normal limits. Her only complaints are slight nausea in the mornings, breast tenderness, and mild fatigue. Her pelvic exam reveals a platypelloid pelvis (Figure 1.1) with arch >90° and flat sacrum, uterus enlarged to 5- to 6-week size, and slight tenderness in right ovarian area. All of her prenatal labs are wnl.

Case Study

She calls the clinic two weeks after her initial visit complaining of spotting. The breast tenderness, nausea, and fatigue have gotten worse. Upon exam, her cervix is closed and the uterus is approximately 6- to 8-week size. Chadwick's sign is positive. No fetal heart tones can be located by Doppler. A small amount of dark blood is seen at the cervical os.

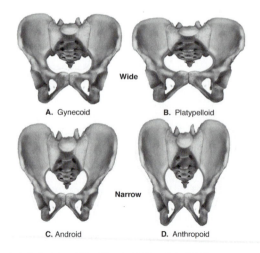

Figure 1.1 *Female pelvic types. The platypelloid pelvis (B) is common among Asian women*

Questions

1. If today's date is March 10 and her last normal menstrual period (LNMP) was January 31, what is her due date? (She has regular 28-day cycles.)

2. How many weeks pregnant is she today?

3. What is the significance of her pelvic structure?

4. What is Chadwick's sign?

5. What are the underlying causes of the breast tenderness and fatigue?

6. Nausea and vomiting in pregnancy are common. When would they not be considered normal? What advice can the nurse give Allyson to relieve her nausea and vomiting?

7. What are the primary causes of the nausea and vomiting in early pregnancy?

8. List three questions the nurse needs to ask Allyson relating to the spotting?

9. Why is it important that the nurse listen to Allyson and respond to her in a therapeutic manner rather than a reassuring manner?

10. Give at least five possible causes for the bleeding.

11. Give three possible explanations for the tenderness in the right ovarian area.

12. When can Allyson expect the early symptoms of discomfort to begin to get better?

13. What advice should the nurse give Allyson regarding the bleeding?

14. What is the significance that fetal heart tones have not been heard?

15. What screening/diagnostic tests should be ordered at this time?

Questions and Suggested Answers

1. If today's date is March 10 and her LNMP was January 31, what is her due date? (She has regular 28-day cycles.) Her due date is November 7.

2. How many weeks pregnant is she today? She is six weeks pregnant.

3. What is the significance of her pelvic structure? A platypelloid pelvis is common in Asian women. A platypelloid pelvis has a short anterior–posterior diameter and wide transverse diameter. Labor often has a delay at the inlet, and a cesarean section is often necessary due to the inability of the fetal head to navigate through the pelvis. This is called cephalopelvic disproportion (CPD). Encouraging and assisting these women to push in squatting positions can make delivery easier.

4. What is Chadwick's sign? Chadwick's sign is a purplish to bluish coloring of the vaginal mucosa, cervix, and vulva that occurs in pregnancy due to the increased blood flow to these areas. This usually occurs by eight weeks gestation. It is considered a presumptive sign of pregnancy in women who are pregnant for the first time (primigravidas).

5. What are the underlying causes of the breast tenderness and fatigue? Estrogen and progesterone increase with pregnancy and can result in discomforts such as these. Breast changes influenced by estrogen may cause tenderness. In early pregnancy the basal metabolic rate (BMR) falls, resulting in fatigue.

6. Nausea and vomiting in pregnancy are common. When would they not be considered normal? When the vomiting is so severe that a woman begins to experience dehydration and electrolyte imbalances, the condition is called hyperemesis gravidarum, and it is a serious complication that needs immediate medical attention and hospitalization. **What advice can the nurse give Allyson to relieve her nausea and vomiting?** The nurse should advise her to eat small, frequent meals that are high in carbohydrates. Sea bands on the wrist, and drinking ginger tea (in moderation) and carbonated ginger ale, which contains real ginger, may be helpful. Vitamin B_6 10 to 25 mg, 3 to 4 times a day may be helpful. In severe cases the clinician may order antiemetics such as promethazine (Phenergan) or prochlorperazine (Compazine). These can be given orally or, if she cannot tolerate oral medications, they may be given rectally.

7. What are the primary causes of the nausea and vomiting in early pregnancy? Maternal sensitivity to the increasing levels of human chorionic gonadotropin (hCG), produced in the placenta, is thought to cause the nausea and vomiting. Hypoglycemia makes the nausea and vomiting worse. Even though as many as 50% of pregnant women normally suffer from nausea and vomiting, the nurse still needs to be aware that in a few cases it can indicate a significant problem. Hyperemesis gravidarum, bulimia, food poisoning, flu, gastroenteritis, hepatitis, intestinal parasites, migraines, pyelonephritis, and appendicitis are also possible reasons why pregnant women vomit.

8. List three questions the nurse needs to ask Allyson related to the spotting?

■ *To identify possible causes:* Did you have intercourse last night? This could indicate trauma. There is increased vascularity in the vaginal area and increased fragility of the small blood vessels. This can cause some spotting with even normal intercourse or vaginal exams. Are you having any other vaginal discharge? Inflammation of the cervix (cervicitis) from vaginal infections may cause spotting.

■ *To assess the amount of bleeding:* Are you still bleeding? How much bleeding have you had? How many pads did you use this morning, and how soaked were they?

■ *To assess the character of the bleeding and associated symptoms:* Have you had any cramping with the spotting? Are you passing any clots? Are you experiencing any backache, fever, or chills? This could indicate a threatened abortion. A backache may be a sign of a urinary tract infection, and the blood could be from the urethra, not the vagina.

9. Why is it important that the nurse listen to Allyson and respond to her in a therapeutic manner rather than a reassuring manner? Many women experience pregnancy losses in the first trimester. Allyson may have many fears about this possibility, and from her obstetrical history, they are well founded. She needs the opportunity to talk about these concerns and have her questions answered as best they can be at this time. Reassurance only closes communication. Once the bleeding stops and a viable pregnancy is established, the nurse can tell her that bleeding such as she experienced at this time in the pregnancy does not necessarily mean that she will be at a higher risk for loss later in the pregnancy.

10. Give at least five possible causes for the bleeding.

■ Implantation bleeding
■ Intercourse or other trauma
■ Potential spontaneous abortion
■ Ectopic pregnancy
■ Trophoblastic disease
■ Cervicitis
■ Hemorrhagic cystitis or pyelonephritis (bleeding from the urethra confused for vaginal bleeding)
■ Cervical polyp
■ Hemorrhoids (rectal bleeding confused for vaginal bleeding)
■ Cervical cancer (least likely)

11. Give three possible explanations for the tenderness in the right ovarian area.

■ Ovarian cyst (corpus luteum)
■ Pulled round ligament
■ Ectopic pregnancy

12. When can Allyson expect the early symptoms of discomfort to begin to get better? Early discomforts will usually subside by the 13th to 15th week of pregnancy when the hCG levels begin to fall.

13. What advice should the nurse give Allyson regarding the bleeding? Pelvic rest should be advised. This constitutes no intercourse or sexual activities that would result in orgasm. She may wish to reduce her overall activity level. Although there is no evidence that if she were aborting this would make any difference, it may make her feel better. She should also avoid breast stimulation at this time since this may stimulate contractions.

14. What is the significance that fetal heart tones have not been heard? This is still early; and although they may be heard by the 8th to 9th week, it is common not to be able to hear them at this time. The fact that her signs and symptoms are getting worse is reassuring since it usually means that the hCG levels are rising, which is consistent with a viable intrauterine pregnancy (IUP). When there is spotting, these signs decrease, and there are no discernable fetal heart tones (FHT), the pregnancy must be evaluated for viability or the possibility of an ectopic pregnancy. An ultrasound can determine both implantation site of the pregnancy and viability. Serial quantitative hCG levels can be used to determine viability. These levels should double every two days. Low levels and slowly increasing levels may indicate ectopic pregnancy. Falling levels indicate a pregnancy loss. The fetal heart movement can be identified by an ultrasound.

15. What screening/diagnostic tests should be ordered at this time? Digital and speculum exam would be appropriate to assess the condition of the cervix, to determine where the bleeding is coming from, and to obtain specimens for cultures and wet mount examination. (After the first trimester a digit exam is never done for bleeding of unknown cause since later it can disrupt a low-lying placenta.) An ultrasound should be ordered to confirm an intrauterine, viable pregnancy and to r/o ectopic pregnancy. Quantitative serial hCG levels may also be ordered.

References

Littleton, L., & Engebretson, J. C. (2002). *Maternal, neonatal, and women's health nursing.* Clifton Park, NY, Thomson Delmar Learning.

Wheeler, L. (2002). *Nurse-midwifery handbook* (2nd ed.). Philadelphia: Lippincott, Williams & Wilkins.

CASE STUDY 3

June

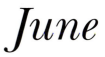

AGE

37

SETTING

- Midwifery prenatal clinic

CULTURAL CONSIDERATIONS

- Orthodox Jewish culture

ETHNICITY

- Jewish American

PRE-EXISTING CONDITION

- AMA

CO-EXISTING CONDITION/CURRENT PROBLEM

- Multiple gestation

COMMUNICATIONS

DISABILITY

SOCIOECONOMIC STATUS

SPIRITUAL/RELIGIOUS

- Orthodox Jewish

PSYCHOSOCIAL

- Close extended family

LEGAL

ETHICAL

PRIORITIZATION

DELEGATION

PHARMACOLOGIC

ALTERNATIVE THERAPY

SIGNIFICANT HISTORY

- Grand multigravida; closely spaced pregnancies

MODERATE

PRENATAL

Level of difficulty: Moderate

Overview: Requires identification of factors that place a multigestational pregnancy at risk. Describes fetal assessment tests. Requires critical thinking to modify teaching to meet the needs of the woman pregnant with multiples.

Client Profile

June is a 37-year-old, G7P6006. This is an unexpected pregnancy. June is an Orthodox Jew. She lives close to both her family and her husband's family. They are a very close family. June home-schools her children, and although she was not expecting this pregnancy, she is fine with it. Her youngest child just turned 15 months old. June started her prenatal care at 10 weeks gestation. She chose a midwife because all of her children have been born at home with a midwife in attendance. She loves the personal care she receives. June values her privacy from strangers, but draws strength and comfort from being surrounded by her extended family. She is five foot three inches tall, and her pre-pregnant weight was 128 pounds. She is certain that her LNMP was June 12. Her cycles are 28 days. She breastfeeds all of her babies for at least one year.

Case Study

At today's visit June is 14 weeks gestation. The midwife finds the following:

- FHT 140 LLQ
- BP 130/78 (initial BP was 128/80)
- FH 1 cm below umbilicus
- FM not felt yet
- Nausea and vomiting several times a day
- Mild headaches several times a week
- Bilateral lower extremity edema +1
- Weight 142 pounds, a gain of 8 pounds in last four weeks

The midwife sends her for an ultrasound to confirm her due date and to rule out multiple gestations. She is diagnosed with twins.

Questions

1. Why did the midwife question her due date or possible multiple gestation at this visit?

2. What nutritional advice should the nurse give June in light of her twin pregnancy?

3. Identify at least four risks that increase with multiple gestations.

4. The midwife explains that June will now need special antepartum care, including being seen by a perinatologist. June tells the nurse that this is not acceptable to her. She feels that all of her pregnancies have been normal and does not want to do anything different this time. How can the nurse help June to obtain care that is safe and acceptable?

5. How does this diagnosis impact June's plans for a home birth?

6. How will June's pregnancy be monitored now that she has been diagnosed with twins?

7. June asks the nurse if the babies will be identical or fraternal twins. How should the nurse respond?

8. Are these babies at any higher risk of anomalies?

9. What steps will be taken to reduce the risk of preterm labor?

10. At 37 weeks gestation June goes into labor. Both babies are in a vertex presentation. The perinatologist has agreed to attempt a vaginal birth. How can the nurse prepare June for her birth?

Questions and Suggested Answers

1. Why did the midwife question her due date and or possible multiple gestation at this visit? Her fundal height is high for her dates.

2. What nutritional advice should the nurse give June in light of her twin pregnancy? A woman carrying twins needs at least 2700 calories a day. June will need extra iron, folic acid, and a diet high in calories, carbohydrates, vitamins, and minerals. If she is put on magnesium sulfate tocolysis and bed rest to prevent preterm labor, she will also need extra calcium. She will need extra fluids.

3. Identify at least four risks that increase with multiple gestations. She is at risk for hyperemesis gravidarum due to the increased levels of hCG, hypertension (both PIH and preeclampsia), gestational diabetes, and preterm labor and birth. Other problems she is at risk for include:

- Cardiopulmonary complications such as pulmonary edema and complications of tocolysis (should it become necessary to stop preterm labor)
- Acute fatty liver of pregnancy
- Gall bladder problems
- Antepartum hemorrhage related to abruption placenta and uterine rupture
- Postpartum hemorrhage and infections

4. The midwife explains that June will now need special antepartum care, including being seen by a perinatologist. June tells the nurse that this is not acceptable to her. She feels that all of her pregnancies have been normal and does not want to do anything different this time. How can the nurse help June to obtain care that is safe and acceptable? Initially, the nurse needs to listen to June and help her determine what it is about the special care that she finds uncomfortable. Considering June's culture and religious beliefs, the nurse should be aware that June is not comfortable with male providers and that she does not like to expand her circle of outside contacts. The nurse may identify a female perinatologist who could possibly be more acceptable to June. The nurse should also find a perinatologist who is comfortable with home birth and midwives so that there will not be a conflict of beliefs between the MD and June. Although June will no longer be a candidate for a home birth, a perinatologist who recognizes this desire is more likely to be able to discuss special care with June in terms that are acceptable to her. June needs respect for her past decisions and choices in care. When mutual respect occurs, it is easier for a client to accept changes in her plans for care. In addition, a perinatologist who respects home birth is more likely to work with the midwife in a collaborative agreement, allowing June to maintain some of the initial plans for her pregnancy. If the nurse has a good rapport with June, she may offer to go to the first perinatologist visit with her, or she may suggest that her mother or mother-in-law accompany her. Ideally, the midwife will be credentialed at the hospital and/or be able to enter into a collaborative management arrangement with the perinatologist and therefore be able to continue in June's care.

5. How does this diagnosis impact June's plans for a home birth? June is no longer a safe candidate for home birth. The nurse can become a liaison for June with the hospital staff. Together they can identify those aspects of home birth that are critical to June. These aspects can then be incorporated, as much as possible, into a hospital birth. The diagnosis of twins does not necessarily mean a cesarean section.

6. How will June's pregnancy be monitored now that she has been diagnosed with twins? June should be seen at least weekly. By 20 weeks she will probably be put on antepartal home monitoring for contractions. She will be taught how to do kick counts as soon as the fetal movements are easily felt. At 26 to 28 weeks, a weekly non-stress test (NST) will be done. This test is used to assess fetal well-being. It evaluates the fetal ability to change her heart rate to meet the need for more oxygen when movement occurs. When the fetus repeatedly increases her heart rate by at least 15 beats per minute for at least 15 seconds when she moves, the test is considered reactive, and it reflects fetal well-being. Both babies will be evaluated. Her hemoglobin will be checked at each visit since women carrying twin pregnancies are at a higher risk for anemia. In addition, since she is a gravida 7 and her last baby is only 15 months old, her iron stores are probably depleted. She will have frequent ultrasounds to compare the fetal growth patterns for both babies. Sometimes, in twin pregnancies one baby will thrive at the expense of the other baby. She will probably have biophysical profiles done weekly after 30 weeks. A biophysical profile includes a series of observations that reflect fetal well-being. These include looking at fetal breathing movements, fetal tone, fetal movement, NST, and the amount of amniotic fluid present. Placenta grading may also be done.

7. June asks the nurse if the babies will be identical or fraternal twins. How should the nurse respond? If the ultrasound shows two separate placentas, then it is clear that the babies are fraternal. However, two separate placentas may fuse and appear as one, which can make it difficult to tell prior to the birth. If there is circulation between the placentas (amnion and chorion are shared), then the babies are identical. Usually this is determined upon the examination of the placentas after birth.

8. Are these babies at any higher risk of anomalies? Yes. The rate of chromosomal anomalies in dizygotic twins is twice that of singleton babies. Monozygotic twins have even higher rates of congenital anomalies. One of the monozygotic twins may be missing a heart or have kidneys that do not function. Placental anomalies are also more common in twin pregnancies.

9. What steps will be taken to reduce the risk of preterm labor? June will be encouraged to maintain a healthy diet and good hydration. She will be taught signs of preterm labor and encouraged to contact her care providers at the earliest signs. She will be carefully monitored for urinary tract or vaginal infections and treated promptly. She will be encouraged to reduce her activities, although bed rest may not be necessary.

10. At 37 weeks gestation June goes into labor. Both babies are in a vertex presentation (Figure 1.2). The perinatologist has agreed to attempt a vaginal birth. How can the nurse prepare June for her birth? After the birth of the first twin the physician may have to use external pressure to direct the second baby into the proper position. Although this is common in all vaginal twin births, this is even more likely because this is June's seventh pregnancy and she probably lacks good abdominal muscle tone. June may find this uncomfortable, and being aware of it ahead of time will help her deal with the discomfort and be able to cooperate.

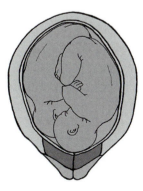

Figure 1.2 *The vertex presentation in multiple gestations*

References

Blackburn, S. (2003). *Maternal, fetal, and neonatal physiology* (2nd ed.). St. Louis, MO: W. B. Saunders Co.

Simpson, K. R., & Creehan, P. A. (2001). *AWHONN perinatal nursing* (2nd ed.). Philadelphia: Lippincott, Williams & Wilkins.

Rana

AGE

26

SETTING

- Private OB setting

CULTURAL CONSIDERATIONS

- Muslim tradition

ETHNICITY

- Middle Eastern

PRE-EXISTING CONDITION

- Low BMI

CO-EXISTING CONDITION/CURRENT PROBLEM

- S < D; closely spaced children; initial low weight and low weight gain

COMMUNICATIONS

DISABILITY

SOCIOECONOMIC STATUS

- Low-middle-class income

SPIRITUAL/RELIGIOUS

- Muslim

PSYCHOSOCIAL

LEGAL

ETHICAL

PRIORITIZATION

DELEGATION

PHARMACOLOGIC

ALTERNATIVE THERAPY

SIGNIFICANT HISTORY

- Multigravida

DIFFICULT

PRENATAL

Level of difficulty: Difficult

Overview: Requires some knowledge of the Muslim culture and early warning signs of developing pre-eclampsia.

Client Profile

Rana is a 26-year-old; G4P3003, married Muslim woman at 26 weeks gestational age. She works as a clerk in a family-run store. This keeps her on her feet for long hours. She is also expected to stock the shelves as needed, which means that she has to bend and lift a lot. At her last prenatal visit (22 weeks) she complained of fatigue, heart burn, lower back pain, and constipation. She keeps the children at the store with her in a back room that is nicely set up as a comfortable lounge with a single bed, TV, and various children's toys. Her children are five, three, and one years old. She just weaned the one-year-old last week. This arrangement works well for her. All in all, she is happy but tired.

Case Study

Rana is five feet six inches tall. Her pre-pregnant weight (PPW) was 106 pounds. Today she is 114 pounds. She lost six pounds in her first trimester due to severe nausea and vomiting. By 15 weeks it was much better and she started to gain weight back. For the past two visits she has been gaining one pound a week. However, she gained six pounds in the last week. Her blood pressure today is 130/76 (IPNV @ 8 wga, her blood pressure was 120/70). Her fundal height is 21 cm; at the last visit it was 2 cm below the umbilicus. The baby is active. The FHT are in the URQ 130 to 140 bpm. Her urine today is +2 protein, + nitrites, and + leukocytes. Because of her religion Rana wears loose clothes that cover her almost completely including her head.

Questions

1. Would the nurse expect Rana's complaints from her last visit to be worse or better at this visit?

2. Discuss Rana's weight and her weight gain/loss pattern. How might this impact her pregnancy?

3. Analyze her blood pressure changes. Are these normal for this period of gestation? If not, why not?

4. How does the fact that Rana wears traditional Muslim clothing make it more difficult to assess her health status at this visit?

5. How can the nurse assess her for edema?

6. What is the significance of the +2 protein in her urine? Give two possible explanations for this.

7. What is the significance of the + nitrites and leukocytes in the urine dip?

8. List three suggestions for Rana to help her at work to reduce the strain on her back.

9. Identify at least three indications that Rana is experiencing a high-risk pregnancy.

10. From the information given, what is your assessment of this baby?

Questions and Suggested Answers

1. Would the nurse expect Rana's complaints from her last visit to be worse or better at this visit? Rana is 26 weeks gestation. At her last visit she complained of fatigue, heart burn, lower back pain, and constipation. These will probably be worse. Many women at this time of pregnancy have more energy and fewer discomforts. However, under the circumstances of her work and three very close pregnancies, Rana is at high risk for anemia, which would account for her increased fatigue. She may complain of symptoms related to a urinary tract infection.

2. Discuss Rana's weight and her weight gain/loss pattern. How might this impact her pregnancy? Rana was very underweight at the beginning of this pregnancy. She was breastfeeding and had a baby under one year old, when she got pregnant. She has probably depleted her stores of essential nutrients. The weight loss in the first trimester is normal, and her current gain back is acceptable in light of her underweight condition and previous loss. However, the six pounds in one week may be a reflection of water retention, which is not normal and needs to be investigated.

3. Analyze her blood pressure changes. Are these normal for this period of gestation? If not, why not? This is not a normal change. At this point in Rana's pregnancy the nurse should expect to see a drop in blood pressure, not a rise. Peripheral resistance is lower due to the influence of progesterone in preparation for the increased blood volume that will soon occur. This should drop her blood pressure at this time. Hypertension is defined as 140/90. Even though her blood pressure is less than this, the increase at this time is a sign that should draw attention. The +2 protein in her urine increases concern over the possibility of her developing significant hypertension.

4. How does the fact that Rana wears traditional Muslim clothing make it more difficult to assess her health status at this visit? The nurse needs to be able to assess the upper body, including the sacral area, hands, and face for signs of edema that are associated with hypertension. Edema limited to lower extremities that occurs at the end of the day is normal and a positive sign of normal vascular volume expansion.

5. How can the nurse assess her for edema? Whenever possible, Rana should be provided with female care providers. The nurse can make sure that Rana's privacy is protected and ask her for permission to examine her arms and lower back. Rana will probably be comfortable removing the extra clothing as long as no men are present.

6. What is the significance of the +2 protein in her urine? Give two possible explanations for this. Plus 2 protein may be associated with decreased kidney perfusion usually associated with hypertension. Increased vaginal contamination may also account for this finding. Serum creatinine and uric acid can be used to further assess the kidneys. Aspartate aminotransferase (AST) assesses kidney and liver involvement. A 24-hour urine test can help determine more accurately the amount of protein being excreted.

7. What is the significance of the + nitrites and leukocytes in the urine dip? These indicate a probable urinary tract infection.

8. List three suggestions for Rana to help her at work to reduce the strain on her back. Do not bend at the waist. She should squat whenever possible to lift objects, such as when she stocks shelves. She should limit standing for long periods of time. Perhaps she can have a chair at the counter of the store. When standing she should use a small block to rest one foot on to shift weight. If she has to lift anything, she should bring it close to her body before trying to lift it. Limit the weight she lifts. Ask for help when she needs it.

9. Identify at least three indications that Rana is experiencing a high-risk pregnancy.

- +2 protein
- Increased BP
- S < D
- 6 pound weight gain in one week

10. From the information given, what is your assessment of this baby? The baby is IUGR (intrauterine growth retardated). This condition seems to have been constant for at least the last four weeks, indicating probably a symmetrical IUGR. This is serious. The baby is at risk of preterm delivery and being born small for gestational age (SGA).

References

Blackburn, S. (2003). *Maternal, fetal, and neonatal physiology* (2nd ed.). St. Louis, MO: W. B. Saunders Co.

Littleton, L., & Engebretson, J. C. (2002). *Maternal, neonatal, and women's health nursing.* Clifton Park, NY: Thomson Delmar Learning.

Wheeler, L. (2002). *Nurse-midwifery handbook* (2nd ed.). Philadelphia: Lippincott, Williams & Wilkins.

Oprah

AGE

16

SETTING

- High school health clinic

CULTURAL CONSIDERATIONS

- Black American impoverished mores

ETHNICITY

- Black American

PRE-EXISTING CONDITION

CO-EXISTING CONDITION/CURRENT PROBLEM

- Headache; elevated BP; epigastric pain; stress

COMMUNICATIONS

DISABILITY

SOCIOECONOMIC STATUS

- Poverty

SPIRITUAL/RELIGIOUS

PSYCHOSOCIAL

- Unstable home; abuse

LEGAL

- Statutory rape

ETHICAL

PRIORITIZATION

DELEGATION

PHARMACOLOGIC

ALTERNATIVE THERAPY

SIGNIFICANT HISTORY

- 2 previous abortions; multigravida

DIFFICULT

PRENATAL

Level of difficulty: Difficult

Overview: Requires that the student be alert for signs of abuse. Requires awareness of risk factors in pregnancy for adolescence. Involves assessing for pre-eclampsia.

Client Profile

Oprah is a 16-year-old; G3P0020, SBF, high school student who lives with her aunt and uncle. She is 28 weeks gestation by LNMP. She has been receiving prenatal care at the school clinic. She has been absent for the past week.

Case Study

Oprah reported to her first hour class this morning complaining of a headache and upper right quadrant pain (URQ). Her teacher sent her to the clinic. The nurse in the clinic checked Oprah's vital signs and obtained the following data:

- T 98.4, P 88; R 18
- BP 136/74 (her normal baseline BP is 118/68.)
- FHT 130s LLQ
- Urine chemstrip. It is positive for ketones and trace protein, otherwise negative.

Oprah told the nurse that she really was ok but did not sleep well last night and was just nervous about a test that she had not studied for. She wanted a chance to rest.

Questions

1. Prior to releasing Oprah to the clinic's quiet room to "just rest," what questions does the nurse need to ask?

2. What further observations does she need to make?

3. Discuss the laws in your area concerning reporting child abuse and statuary rape.

4. What complications is Oprah at risk for related to her age?

5. What is she at risk for related to her gravida/para?

6. What complications is she at risk for due to her race?

7. What is the significance of Oprah's BP, especially as it relates to the pregnancy's gestation?

8. What are the possible sources of the upper right quadrant pain?

9. What is the significance of the findings of positive ketones in her urine?

10. What is the significance of the trace protein?

11. Which of the following actions would be appropriate by the nurse? The nurse should have Oprah:

    a. Rest for 30 minutes and then recheck her BP

    b. Transported to the hospital immediately

    c. Go back to class

    d. Take a Tylenol for her headache. The nurse should scold her for not eating breakfast.

Questions and Suggested Answers

1. Prior to releasing Oprah to the clinic's quiet room to "just rest," what questions does the nurse need to ask?

- Is the baby moving as usual?
- Did she eat breakfast?
- Have her describe the headache:
  - Does she have any vision changes?
  - Have her describe the pain and point to exactly where it hurts.
- Why did she miss school all last week?
- At 16 she has been pregnant three times and has had two abortions. She is missing school and exhibiting signs of stress. She may be an abused child. Even if she is not being abused, she does have psychosocial problems and may be trying to get attention. She needs someone to listen to her and protect her. She needs a social services referral and investigation for possible abuse.

2. What further observations does she need to make?

- Is her abdomen hard and/or tender?
- Does Oprah have any edema, and if so where, and how much?

3. Discuss the laws in your area concerning reporting child abuse and statutory rape. Answers will vary from area to area.

4. What complications is Oprah at risk for related to her age? Her age puts her at risk for pregnancy-induced hypertension/pre-eclampsia.

5. What is she at risk for related to her gravida/para? She has had two abortions; these put her at risk for preterm labor/birth.

6. What complications is she at risk for due to her race? Black women are at a higher risk for chronic hypertension, pregnancy-induced hypertension, pre-eclampsia, preterm labor and birth, and diabetes.

7. What is the significance of Oprah's BP, especially as it relates to the pregnancy's gestation? Her blood pressure at 28 weeks should be slightly below her pre-pregnant BP due to decreased vascular resistance. Her diastolic is slightly elevated but not significantly; however, her systolic is elevated. This may be due to stress and needs to be rechecked after she has rested.

8. What are the possible sources of the upper right quadrant pain? This may have several possible explanations. She may have pain from the baby kicking, it could be gall stones, or it could be liver tenderness related to the hypertension.

9. What is the significance of the findings of positive ketones in her urine? This is a sign of fasting. It may give a reason for her headache since hypoglycemia may cause headaches.

10. What is the significance of the trace protein? This may have several sources. It could be normal, reflecting an increase in the excreted protein during pregnancy due to increased GFR when the protein-filtered load exceeds the tubular capacity to reabsorb the protein. It could be contamination from a normal vaginal discharge (leucorrhoea), or it could be related to poor kidney function as a result of poor perfusion if she has hypertension.

11. Which of the following actions would be appropriate by the nurse? The nurse should have Oprah:

    a. Rest for 30 minutes and then recheck her BP

References

Blackburn, S. (2003). *Maternal, fetal, and neonatal physiology* (2nd ed.). St. Louis, MO: W. B. Saunders Co.

Littleton, L., & Engebretson, J. C. (2002). *Maternal, neonatal, and women's health nursing.* Clifton Park, NY: Thomson Delmar Learning.

Wheeler, L. (2002). *Nurse-midwifery handbook* (2nd ed.). Philadelphia: Lippincott, Williams & Wilkins.

Alina

AGE

- 22

SETTING

- Prenatal clinic

CULTURAL CONSIDERATIONS

- Dominican Republican traditions

ETHNICITY

- Black/Caribbean Islander

PRE-EXISTING CONDITION

CO-EXISTING CONDITION/CURRENT PROBLEM

- Placenta previa

COMMUNICATIONS

DISABILITY

SOCIOECONOMIC STATUS

- Upper middle class

SPIRITUAL/RELIGIOUS

PSYCHOSOCIAL

- Divides her time between two countries; single parent

LEGAL

ETHICAL

PRIORITIZATION

DELEGATION

PHARMACOLOGIC

- Methylergonovine maleate (Methergine); Hemabate; oxytocin (Pitocin)

ALTERNATIVE THERAPY

SIGNIFICANT HISTORY

- Mulitgravida

ANTEPARTUM through postpartum

Level of difficulty: Difficult

Overview: Requires recognition of a placenta previa and the implications for care including higher risk for postpartum hemorrhage. Discussion of types of cesarean section and VBAC.

Client Profile

Alina is a 22-year-old, SBF who recently emigrated from the Dominican Republic. She is a G2P0101 currently at 28 wga. Alina started prenatal care at 12 weeks gestation. She is five feet seven inches tall, and her current weight is 140 pounds. She is a strikingly beautiful model and the only visible signs of her pregnancy thus far are enlarged breasts and a small abdominal pouch only visible from the front. Her total weight gain thus far is 10 pounds. She only eats raw vegetables, drinks protein shakes, and exercises at least a full hour every day. Her mother "back home" in the Dominican Republic is raising her first baby. She plans to either send this baby to her mother, or if she can, she would like to try to bring her daughter and mother to the United States to stay with her. She plans a home birth at her apartment.

Case Study

Alina is being seen today at the prenatal clinic because of a complaint of decreased fetal movement and a bloody discharge.

Questions

1. When Alina called regarding the decreased movement and blood discharge, what questions should the nurse have asked?

2. Although this is not a regular prenatal visit, what assessments will be made?

3. Will a vaginal exam be done? If so describe it.

4. What assessment tests will be ordered?

5. What are the usual causes of bleeding at 28 weeks gestation?

6. The ultrasound reveals a placenta previa. The bleeding has stopped. How will this affect Alina's plans for delivery?

7. Alina is devastated. She models swimsuits and is sure that a cesarean section will ruin her career. How should the nurse respond?

8. At 38 weeks the baby is breech and the bleeding has started again. A cesarean section is done and the baby's APGARS are 9-9. Alina is doing well until 30 minutes after the delivery in recovery she begins a profuse hemorrhage. Give possible explanations for the bleeding.

9. Give at least three immediate nursing actions appropriate at this time.

10. Alina loses approximately 2000 mL of blood prior to the bleeding being stopped. How might this affect her recovery? (Her hemocrit at 24 hours is 29%.)

Questions and Suggested Answers

1. When Alina called regarding the decreased movement and blood discharge, what questions should the nurse have asked?

- Are you currently bleeding?
- How much? Are you using a pad? If so have you had to change it? If yes, how often? What color is the blood? Are there clots? This is a rough attempt to distinguish the amount of blood loss and the character.
- Are you also having cramping or any other type of pain? If so describe it. This may help determine if the bleeding is possibly previa, abruption, or bloody show as in preterm labor.
- Did you have intercourse in the last 24 hours? Trauma may cause spotting.
- Are you having any other vaginal discharge (color, odor, itching)? Cervicitis may cause spotting.
- How many movements have you felt in the last 4 to 6 hours?
- When did you eat last? (Babies sometimes have decreased movements when the mother is hypoglycemic.)
- Are you feeling faint, anxious, or nauseated? (Excessive bleeding can cause these symptoms, and the bleeding may be hidden as in placenta abruption.)

2. Although this is not a regular prenatal visit, what assessments will be made?

- Maternal vital signs and BP
- Fundal height
- Assessment of the abdomen (Is it hard and/or board-like?)
- Is her abdomen tender?
- FHT
- Urine chemstrip analysis
- Check for edema
- Ask about vision changes and/or headaches
- Ask about signs of UTI
- Fetal movement

3. Will a vaginal exam be done? If so, describe it. A digital exam should not be done until a previa can be ruled out with an ultrasound. A sterile speculum exam can be done to observe the cervix for cervicitis and to obtain specimens for culture if history and inspection indicate the need.

4. What assessment tests will be ordered? Ultrasound and vaginal and urine cultures are appropriate.

5. What are the usual causes of bleeding at 28 weeks gestation? Placenta previa and abruption must be ruled out. The most common causes of bleeding in the second trimester are cervicitis and slight trauma from intercourse or vaginal exam.

6. The ultrasound reveals a placenta previa (Figure 1.3). The bleeding has stopped. How will this affect Alina's plans for delivery? She will need a cesarean section at the hospital.

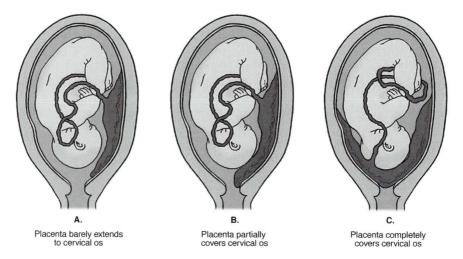

A.
Placenta barely extends
to cervical os

B.
Placenta partially
covers cervical os

C.
Placenta completely
covers cervical os

Figure 1.3 *Three types of placenta previa: (A) Low implantation (marginal), (B) Partial placenta previa, (C). Total placenta previa*

7. Alina is devastated. She models swimsuits and is sure that a cesarean section will ruin her career. How should the nurse respond? Unless the low position of the placenta prevents using it, the most commonly used technique, a lower segment transverse incision through the uterus for cesarean section, will allow the skin incision to be low, just under the pubic hairline. This should heal without a visible scar. If the placenta is located more on the posterior wall of the uterus, the obstetrician may be able to do a low segment transverse incision into the uterus, which will possibly increase her chances to have a vaginal birth the next pregnancy (VBAC).

8. At 38 weeks the baby is breech and the bleeding has started again. A cesarean section is done and the baby's APGARS are 9-9. Alina is doing well until 30 minutes after the delivery. In recovery she begins a profuse hemorrhage. Give possible explanations for the bleeding. Even with a well-contracted uterus, the lower segment does not contract as well as the upper segment. Since she had a placenta previa, which places the placenta in the lower part of the uterus, once it separates from the uterine wall it is difficult for the contracting uterus to constrict these now exposed vessels.

9. Give at least three immediate nursing actions appropriate at this time.

■ Check her uterus to see if it is firm. Even a well-contracted uterus may not be able to stop bleeding from the placental site if the site is in the lower segment (as it is in the previa). Massage if boggy.
■ Notify OB stat.
■ Be sure an IV is patent and add oxytocin if there is a standing order. Be prepared to give methylergonovine maleate (Methergine), if she is not

hypertensive, or Hemabate if she does not have a history of asthma and it is ordered.

■ Start a second IV with ringers lactate. Use a large bore catheter in case a blood transfusion is needed.

■ Be prepared to move the mother back to the delivery room or to an operating room as soon as the physician is ready.

10. Alina loses approximately 2000 mL of blood prior to the bleeding being stopped. How might this affect her recovery? (Her hematocrit at 24 hours is 29%.) She will be at risk for infection, will be very fatigued, and may find her emotional recovery more difficult as a result of the fatigue. She will need iron supplementation and a diet high in iron; she may not need a transfusion. Fatigue may interfere with breastfeeding and her ability to care for the newborn. In some cases of severe postpartum hemorrhage, the pituitary gland may become damaged, which will interfere with milk production. This is called Sheehan's syndrome. It will usually not manifest itself unless the blood loss is so severe that the woman goes into shock. Sheehan's syndrome may also cause the loss of pubic and axillary hair.

Reference

Cunningham, F. G., et al. (1993). *Williams Obstetrics* (19th ed.). Norwalk, CT: Appleton & Lange.

Bess

AGE	**SPIRITUAL/RELIGIOUS**
32	■ Catholic
SETTING	**PSYCHOSOCIAL**
■ Client's home	
CULTURAL CONSIDERATIONS	**LEGAL**
■ Hispanic American culture	
ETHNICITY	**ETHICAL**
■ Hispanic American second-generation	
PRE-EXISTING CONDITION	**PRIORITIZATION**
CO-EXISTING CONDITION/CURRENT PROBLEM	**DELEGATION**
■ Hyperemesis gravidarum	
COMMUNICATIONS	**PHARMACOLOGIC**
	■ Promethazine (Phenergan)
DISABILITY	**ALTERNATIVE THERAPY**
	SIGNIFICANT HISTORY
SOCIOECONOMIC STATUS	■ Primigravida

ANTEPARTUM

Level of difficulty: Difficult

Overview: Requires that the student be able to identify the effects of pregnancy on a woman's immune system, understand nutritional needs of pregnancy and the effects of malnutrition, and be able to assess and identify the signs of infection with a central line.

Client Profile

Bess is a 32-year-old, G1P0, MHF at 24 wga. Bess's grandparents immigrated to Miami, Florida, before her parents were born. Even though she is a second-generation Hispanic American, she has spent her whole life in a very Hispanic environment. Her medical, surgical, and family histories are all benign. Bess is five feet five inches, and her pre-pregnant weight was 103 pounds. She has been experiencing severe nausea and vomiting that has gotten worse over the past two weeks. She was hospitalized and put on IV hydration and sedation for 24 hours. The nausea and vomiting continue. She has lost 15 pounds in the past two weeks, and this makes her current weight 106 pounds. Her obstetrician started her on promethazine (Phenergan) suppositories and total parenteral nutrition (TPN) with a central venous catheter (CVC). She is sent home at her and her family's request, with the CVC and home health care to follow up with daily TPN.

Case Study

Bess has been on home health care and daily TPN for three weeks. The baby is continuing to grow, and her fundal height is appropriate for size. The nausea and vomiting have subsided; however, every time she attempts to eat again it reoccurs, therefore she has been kept NPO with all of her nutrition and fluids being provided through IV and TPN. The home health nurse checks on Bess at least once a day, sets up the TPN, and monitors the site as well as educates the family on her care.

Questions

1. Make a list of the possible problems that can occur with TPN being administered through a CVC.

2. What is the etiology of hyperemesis gravidarum?

3. How does the pregnancy affect Bess's risk for infection?

4. List four signs of infection that the home health nurse needs to be alert for.

5. At 27 weeks gestation, Bess complains of swollen feet. How should the home health nurse react to this symptom?

6. Discuss the pros and cons of home heath care for this client.

7. What labs would the nurse anticipate will be required for Bess on a regular basis?

8. Bess's CBC comes back with the following results:

H&H 10.8 g/dL & 31%
RBC 4.5 M/ml
WBC 10.5 K/ml
MCV 80 fL
MCH 27 pg
MCHC 32 g/dL
Platelet count 146,000/mL
Neutrophils 72%
Lymphocytes 20%
Monocytes 6%
Eosinophils 1%
Bassophils 1%

What is the significance of these findings?

9. How often should the home health nurse change the CVC dressing? Outline the specific technique for changing it.

10. At 30 weeks, Bess asks her nurse how much longer it will be before her obstetrician can just take the baby. She is tired of being pregnant and so sick. What is the most appropriate answer by the nurse?

Questions and Suggested Answers

1. Make a list of the possible problems that can occur with TPN being administered through a CVC. Problems that can arise from total parenteral nutrition include risk from infection, risk of thrombus formation, risk of fluid and electrolyte imbalance, risk of glucose imbalance and bone demineralization, fatty liver, dehydration, fluid overload, and acid/base imbalance. Catheter complications include those associated with placement and infection.

2. What is the etiology of hyperemesis gravidarum? The etiology of hyperemesis gravidarum is unknown; however, there does seem to be some connection between high levels of hCG and hyperemesis gravidarum. For example, there is increased risk when a molar pregnancy or multiple gestations exists. The hCG levels are very high in both of these conditions. Hyperemesis gravidarum may also be associated with high stress.

3. How does the pregnancy affect Bess's risk for infection? Pregnancy reduces a woman's immune response. If it did not, she would be at risk of rejecting the fetus because the fetal genetic makeup is different from that of the mother.

4. List four signs of infection that the home health nurse needs to be alert for. Four signs are fever, chills, malaise, and elevated white blood count. If the catheter were infected the site may not show any signs of infection. If the site was infected, then redness, warmth, and heat at the site would indicate infection and possible thrombus.

5. At 27 weeks gestation, Bess complains of swollen feet. How should the home health nurse react to this symptom? At 27 weeks gestation, dependent edema may be associated with normal pregnancy. Dependent edema will not be present when the woman first arises and disappears after elevating her feet. However, the nurse needs to be alert for generalized edema and upper-body edema and, if present, determine whether there is any possible connection between these symptoms and the CVC line placement, infection, and problems related to TPN.

6. Discuss the pros and cons of home health care for this client. Disadvantages of home health care for this client include risk for poor communication between team members, possibly slower response time from the home health agency and/or the physician, delay in getting lab reports to the physician, and difficulty in keeping supplies including TPN solution available. Pros include keeping the mother out of an environment that carries high risk for infections, comforting the mother by allowing her to be in her own home, and causing less disturbance of the family unit. Home care may be more culturally acceptable to Bess.

7. What labs would the nurse anticipate will be required for Bess on a regular basis? Bess will need to have her fluid and electrolytes monitored, her blood sugar monitored, and frequent CBCs to monitor for infection.

8. Bess's CBC comes back with the following results:

H&H 10.8 g/dL & 31%
RBC 4.5 M/ml
WBC 10.5 K/ml
MCV 80 fL
MCH 27 pg
MCHC 32 g/dL
Platelet count 146,000/mL
Neutrophils 72%
Lymphocytes 20%
Monocytes 6%
Eosinophils 1%
Bassophils 1%

What is the significance of these findings? This CBC reflects essentially normal levels with slight anemia.

9. How often should the home health nurse change the CVC dressing? Outline the specific technique for changing it. The dressing needs to be changed whenever the integrity of the dressing is questioned, becomes wet, or in any way appears to not provide a sterile protection of the site. Additionally, a regular changing of the dressing should be done at least once a week. Too frequent changing can damage the skin around the catheter and actually increase infection. The dressing needs to be changed under sterile conditions. This includes having the mother as well as the nurse wear a mask during the change.

10. At 30 weeks, Bess asks her nurse how much longer it will be before her obstetrician can just take the baby. She is tired of being pregnant and so sick. What is the most appropriate answer by the nurse? As long as the baby is growing properly and the mother's and baby's health is being preserved through the TPN, it is best to allow the baby to continue to grow a few more weeks. At around 35 weeks, the obstetrician may do an amniocentesis to check to see if the baby's lungs are mature. Once the baby has reached that point of development that his or her lungs can function well on their own, it is safe to induce the labor and deliver the baby.

References

Blackburn, S. (2003). *Maternal, fetal, and neonatal physiology* (2nd ed.). St. Louis, MO: W. B. Saunders Co.

Whitneye, N., Cataldo, C. B., & Rolfer, S. R. (2002). *Understanding normal and clinical nutrition.* Belmont, CA: Thompson/Wadsworth Learning.

AGE

28

SETTING

- Public health clinic

CULTURAL CONSIDERATIONS

- Mexican culture; immigrant community

ETHNICITY

- Hispanic

PRE-EXISTING CONDITION

- Obesity; undiagnosed diabetes mellitus

CO-EXISTING CONDITION/CURRENT PROBLEM

COMMUNICATIONS

DISABILITY

SOCIOECONOMIC STATUS

SPIRITUAL/RELIGIOUS

PSYCHOSOCIAL

LEGAL

ETHICAL

PRIORITIZATION

DELEGATION

PHARMACOLOGIC

- Iron supplement

ALTERNATIVE THERAPY

- Yellow dock root with nettle, parsley, and peppermint; dandelion leaf tea

SIGNIFICANT HISTORY

- Multigravida

PRENATAL, second trimester

Level of difficulty: Difficult

Overview: Requires an understanding of Hispanic culture, risk factors associated with this ethnic group, and prenatal screening tests. This case requires an understanding of the hematological changes that occur with pregnancy and identification of signs and symptoms associated with diabetes.

DIFFICULT

Client Profile

Del is a 23-year-old, recent Mexican immigrant. She works as a manager at a large import/export business. Del is a G2P0101. She was 22 weeks gestational age (wga) at her initial prenatal visit. She is obese. She is married. Her first child, a boy, was born in Mexico via a normal spontaneous vaginal delivery (NSVD) and is now three years old.

Case Study

This is Del's second prenatal visit. Her first visit was four weeks ago. She complains of fatigue, hemorrhoids, and mild headaches. The nurse reviews Del's lab work from her initial visit to go over it with Del and finds the following: Blood type A positive, antibody screen negative, hemoglobin of 10.2 g/dL and hematocrit of 31% (indices wnl), urinalysis wnl, urine culture negative, all STI screens negative, rubella 1:18 (lab reference level is 1:16 and higher is immune), blood glucose 1-hour screen was 148, PAP wnl, quad screen—no increased risk, and ultrasound indicates the fetus is large for gestational age. Her fundal height is 29 cm. The FHT are 140s in the LLQ. She has no edema. Her BP is 118/78 (the same as at the last visit).

Questions

1. What physical assessments should be made at this visit?

2. How serious is Del's low H&H?

3. What might account for these low levels?

4. What is the significance of Del's 1-hour glucose screen?

5. Are further glucose screening tests needed?

6. If so, which ones?

7. What factors put Del at a higher risk for diabetes?

8. What is the significance of the ultrasound finding of large for gestational age (LGA)?

9. At what point in the pregnancy is glucose screening usually done? Why?

10. Identify at least two nursing diagnoses that would apply if this client is diagnosed with gestational diabetes.

11. Why is the quad screen done, and what are the components tested for in the quad screen?

12. Explain the results of the quad screen.

Questions and Suggested Answers

1. What physical assessments should be made at this visit?

- Fundal height
- Inquire about fetal movement
- BP

- Weight
- Assessment for edema
- Urine chemstrip for ketones, nitrites, leukocytes, glucose, and protein
- Ask about headaches, vision changes, signs and symptoms of UTI

2. How serious is Del's low H&H? This is low normal for this time in the pregnancy.

3. What might account for these low levels? Her low levels are probably related to normal hemodilution, pseudoanemia, or physiologic anemia. She should be encouraged to eat foods high in iron such as dried fruits, dandelion leaf tea, fresh green leafy vegetables, molasses, and whole grains. She should be offered iron supplements and be taught ways to reduce constipation. Other sources of iron include a commercial herbal combination called Floradix. Yellow dock root with nettle, parsley, and peppermint are all good herbal sources for iron.

4. What is the significance of Del's 1-hour glucose screen? This is elevated and may indicate the existence of pregestational diabetes or the development of gestational diabetes.

5. Are further glucose screening tests needed? Yes. Further testing is needed to rule in or rule out diabetes at this time. Del's fundal height is also high for dates (S > D).

6. If so, which ones? A 3-hour glucose tolerance test and possibly an HgbA1c would be appropriate. Two abnormal readings in the 3-hour test will identify diabetes, and the A1c will give a more comprehensive picture, identifying if the hyperglycemia has persisted for a period of several weeks. It identifies the amount of glucose that is permanently bound to hemoglobin and reflects blood sugar levels over the past 4–8 weeks.

7. What factors put Del at a higher risk for diabetes? Del's weight is high for her height. Being a Hispanic American (Mexican) puts her at a higher risk for diabetes but not for gestational diabetes.

8. What is the significance of the ultrasound finding of large for gestational age (LGA)? This may be an indication of pregestational diabetes or gestational diabetes. It could also be a sign of incorrect dates. *Note:* Ultrasound done after 20 wga should not be relied upon for dating a pregnancy if it conflicts with the LNMP confirmed early in the pregnancy.

9. At what point in the pregnancy is glucose screening usually done? Why? Glucose screening is usually done at 26 to 28 weeks when the hPL levels are high and are exhibiting the greatest effect on insulin utilization.

10. Identify at least two nursing diagnoses that would apply if this client is diagnosed with gestational diabetes.

1. Knowledge deficit r/t dietary restriction needed to control blood sugar

2. Anxiety r/t potential fetal risk associated with gestational diabetes.

11. Why is the quad screen done, and what are the components tested for in the quad screen? These tests are also called maternal serum multiple-marker screening (MMS). If the mother has gestational diabetes, the accuracy of the test is less. Del's requisition for the MMS needs to indicate that she is obese and a gestational diabetic. The optimal time for screening is 16 to 18½ weeks gestation. The quad screen is used to identify which fetuses are at risk for open neural tube defects and trisomy. AFP, estriol, hCG, and maternal serum inhibin A are the four components. It's important to note that this is a screening tool and is not diagnostic. False-positive findings are common due to inaccurate due dates.

12. Explain the results of the quad screen. Higher levels of alpha fetoprotein (AFP) indicate a risk for open neural tube defect (ONTD); low levels of AFP with high hCG and low levels of estriol may indicate Down syndrome. Even when the fetus is normal, increased levels of AFP may indicate risks for hypertension, placental anomalies, low birth weight babies, and preterm birth.

References

Gabbe, S., Niebyl, J., & Simpson, J. (2003). *Obstetrics normal & problem pregnancies.* New York: Churchill/Livingstone.

Libster, M. (2002). *Delmar's integrative herb guide for nurses.* Clifton Park, NY: Thomson Delmar Learning.

Morgan, G., & Hamilton, C. (2003). *Practice guidelines for obstetrics and gynecology* (2nd ed.). Philadelphia: Lippincott, Williams & Wilkins.

Simpson, K. R., & Creehan, P. A. (2001). *AWHONN perinatal nursing* (2nd ed.). Philadelphia: Lippincott, Williams & Wilkins.

Tiran, D., & Mack, S. (1995). *Complementary therapies for pregnancy and childbirth.* London: Baillière Tindall.

Wheeler, L. (2002). *Nurse-midwifery handbook* (2nd ed.). Philadelphia: Lippincott, Williams & Wilkins.

Whitney, N., Cataldo, C. B., & Rolfer, S. R. (2002). *Understanding normal and clinical nutrition.* Belmont, CA: Thompson/Wadsworth Learning.

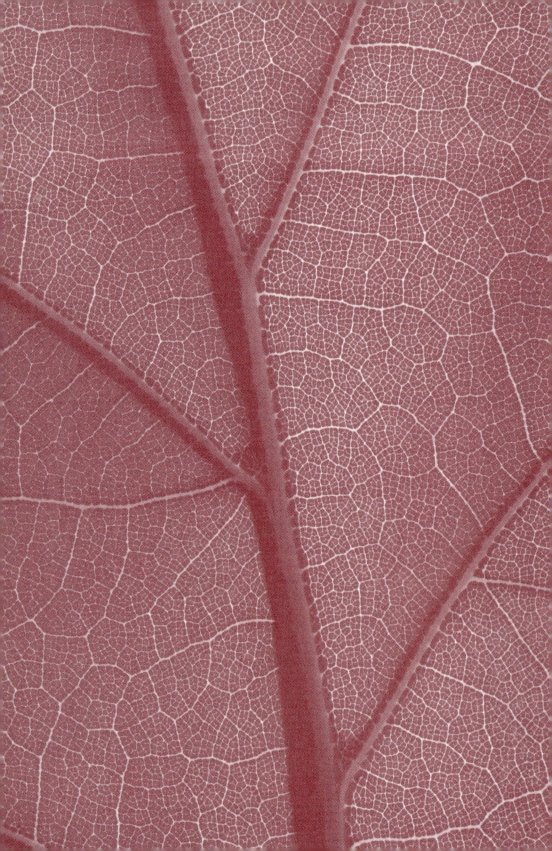

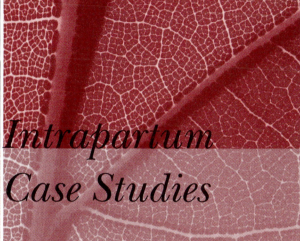

PART TWO

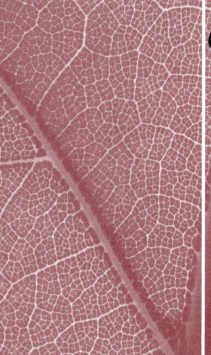

Intrapartum
Case Studies

Ileana

AGE

29

SETTING

- Birth center

CULTURAL CONSIDERATIONS

- Second-generation Cuban immigrant traditions

ETHNICITY

- Hispanic American

PRE-EXISTING CONDITION

- History of preterm birth

CO-EXISTING CONDITION/CURRENT PROBLEM

- Cord compression

COMMUNICATIONS

DISABILITY

SOCIOECONOMIC STATUS

SPIRITUAL/RELIGIOUS

PSYCHOSOCIAL

- Grief due to wrong sex identification on ultrasound

LEGAL

ETHICAL

PRIORITIZATION

DELEGATION

PHARMACOLOGIC

ALTERNATIVE THERAPY

SIGNIFICANT HISTORY

- Multigravida; history of preterm birth

INTRAPARTUM

Level of difficulty: Easy

Overview: This case requires a knowledge base about fetal heart changes during labor. It requires critical thinking to assess and determine appropriate actions for a client experiencing cord compression in labor.

Client Profile

Ileana is a 29-year-old, MHF G3P1102 at 40 wga in active labor at the birth center. Her prenatal course has been uneventful. She gained 22 pounds with this pregnancy. Although she had one previous premature baby, the baby did well and is now three years old. Her husband and sister accompany Ileana in labor. She has two little girls, and the ultrasound done two months ago indicated that this is a baby boy. She is in good spirits and handling her contractions very well.

Case Study

Ileana has been in active labor for six hours. She is 9 cm, 100% effaced, and −2 station. She is returning from the bathroom when her water breaks.

Questions

1. What stage of labor is Ileana in?

2. What is the significance of her being 9 cm dilated, 100% effaced, and −2 station?

3. How does the fact that she is a multipara influence her progress in labor?

4. What is the significance of her water breaking and being −2 station?

5. What is the most important nursing action to be taken at this time?

6. The nurse checks the fetal heart tones and finds them to be 90 bpm. The baseline has been 130 to the 140s. What is the significance of this, and what nursing actions are needed at this time?

7. The fluid is clear and light yellow in color. What is the significance of this?

8. After Ileana is placed on her side, the fetal heart tones return to the baseline of 130–140s. What was the most probable cause of the deceleration?

9. The nurse continues to monitor carefully the next few contractions and notes the following: Baseline 130s with accelerations noted between contractions; average long-term variability; and decelerations mirroring contractions with return to baseline by the end of each contraction. What is the most probable cause of the decelerations?

10. What nursing actions are needed at this time?

11. Ileana states that she has to push. How should the nurse respond?

12. After 20 minutes of pushing Ileana delivers a beautiful baby girl with APGARS of 9 and 10. Ileana and her husband are visibly upset at the sex of the baby and ask, "How can this be? They told us the baby was a boy." Discuss the best way for the nurse to handle this situation.

Questions and Suggested Answers

1. What stage of labor is Ileana in? Ileana is in the active phase of first-stage labor, end of transition.

2. What is the significance of her being 9 cm dilated, 100% effaced, and −2 station? The baby is still high in the pelvis even though she is nearly completely dilated. There is increased risk for cord prolapse when the membranes rupture.

3. How does the fact that she is a multipara influence her progress in labor? Finding the baby still high in a multigravida is not unusual. Had she been a primigravida, this would have been a sign of a possible problem. The better muscle tone in a primigravida will usually direct the baby into the pelvis, encouraging descent earlier in a primigravida than in a multigravida. This is called lightening. When a multigravida does experience lightening early, she may carry the baby very low in her pelvis due to the weaker pelvic support muscles.

4. What is the significance of her water breaking and being −2 station? There is the possibility of prolapsed cord with ruptured membranes and a high presenting part.

5. What is the most important nursing action to be taken at this time? Get her to lie down and check the heart tones of the baby to rule out prolapsed cord.

6. The nurse checks the fetal heart tones and finds them to be 90 bpm. The baseline has been 130 to the 140s. What is the significance of this, and what nursing actions are needed at this time? There may be compression of the umbilical cord. If uncorrected this could compromise the fetus and even result in fetal death. VE is needed to check for prolapsed cord.

7. The fluid is clear and light yellow in color. What is the significance of this? This could indicate light meconium in the fluid. This is usually not a problem in a term infant. Thick meconium can lead to meconium aspiration syndrome in the infant, resulting in pneumonia. After Ileana is placed on her side, the fetal heart tones return to the baseline of 130 to the 140s. Yellow fluid may also indicate infection. Other signs that may indicate an infection are an odor to the fluid and/or a rise in the fetal heart rate baseline and/or maternal temperature.

8. After Ilena is placed on her side, the fetal heart tones return to the baseline of 130–140s. What was the most probable cause of the deceleration? The change in position relieved the pressure on the cord. This supports the theory that it was cord compression.

9. The nurse continues to monitor carefully the next few contractions and notes the following: Baseline 130s with accelerations noted between contractions; average long-term variability; and decelerations mirroring contractions, with return to baseline by the end of each contraction. What is the most probable cause of the decelerations? This is a reassuring pattern of accelerations indicating good fetal response and early decelerations indicating pressure on a descending head with vagal nerve response. The baby has probably descended.

10. What nursing actions are needed at this time? The nurse needs to continue to monitor the mother's vital signs, hydration status, bladder and contractions, relaxation between contractions, and the baby's heart rate.

11. Ileana states that she has to push. How should the nurse respond? Do a vaginal exam to see if she is completely dilated, and if so, encourage her to push. Continue to monitor the baby.

12. After 20 minutes of pushing Ileana delivers a beautiful baby girl with APGARS of 9 and 10. Ileana and her husband are visibly upset at the sex of the baby and ask, "How can this be? They told us the baby was a boy." Discuss the best way for the nurse to handle this situation. The nurse needs to understand that the family may actually have to grieve the loss of their "anticipated son" before they can bond with this new baby. This is their third girl. The Hispanic culture, like many cultures, puts a high value on producing a son. The birth of another daughter may be very disappointing to them when they expected a son. This is one of the dangers of relying on ultrasound to tell the parents the sex of the baby. It is important to stress during the prenatal period that, unless a high-resolution ultrasound has been done with highly skilled operators, parents should always have some degree of doubt about the infant's sex. The nurse needs to allow the couple time to express their loss without being judgmental. It is important that the mother and baby not be separated in order to allow time for bonding. The father should be encouraged to stay with the mother and baby after the delivery so that they can become acquainted with this new arrival since she was unexpected and may seem even more of a stranger to them.

References

Blackburn, S. (2003). *Maternal, fetal, and neonatal physiology* (2nd ed.). Philadelphia: W. B. Saunders Co.

Littleton, L., & Engebretson, J. C. (2002). *Maternal, neonatal, and women's health nursing.* Clifton Park, NY: Thomson Delmar Learning.

Marie

AGE	**SPIRITUAL/RELIGIOUS**
23	■ Catholic/voodoo
SETTING	**PSYCHOSOCIAL**
■ Home	
CULTURAL CONSIDERATIONS	**LEGAL**
■ Recent Haitian immigrant	■ Understanding of OSHA guidelines for home births
ETHNICITY	**ETHICAL**
■ Haitian	
PRE-EXISTING CONDITION	**PRIORITIZATION**
CO-EXISTING CONDITION/CURRENT PROBLEM	**DELEGATION**
COMMUNICATIONS	**PHARMACOLOGIC**
	■ (D) immune globulin vaccination (RhoGAM); oxytocin (Pitocin)
DISABILITY	**ALTERNATIVE THERAPY**
SOCIOECONOMIC STATUS	**SIGNIFICANT HISTORY**
■ Lower middle class	■ Primigravida

MODERATE

INTRAPARTUM

Level of difficulty: Moderate

Overview: The case requires that the student have an understanding of the concepts of sterile technique and OSHA guidelines as they apply in a home delivery. The student is also required to identify how the fetus and the maternal contractions are monitored in an out-of-hospital delivery. Mechanism for delivery of the placenta is discussed.

Client Profile

Marie and her husband Eugene are very excited about the coming birth of their first baby. They came to the States from Haiti six months ago and were pleased to find a Certified Professional Midwife (CPM) to provide prenatal care and assist them to birth their baby at home. Marie has been attending prenatal care at Angle Care Birth Center. This center offers the choice of either birth center delivery or home birth. The home birth team is made up of the CPM, an RN birth assistant, and usually one or two student midwives. Marie and her husband are pleased that they have seen the same individuals throughout the pregnancy, and they made the decision as to which midwife, nurse, and students will be invited to their home birth. Marie's pregnancy has been very normal. Marie gained a total of 26 pounds and started pregnancy at 120 pounds. Her BP at the last visit was 110/68. The baby's growth has been right on schedule with a fundal height at 36 cm at the last visit. Marie eats well, exercises, and has read everything she can get her hands on about labor and birth. Her urine has remained negative throughout the pregnancy. Marie is now 38 weeks gestation. The baby's estimated weight is seven pounds.

Case Study

Eugene called the RN this morning to let her know that Marie had been having contractions all night. This morning they are two minutes apart and lasting a full minute. He sounds anxious as he tells the nurse that she is beginning to have a difficult time getting through the contractions. He has called his mother and her mother to also come over. The RN advises him to stay calm and that the CPM and students will be there within 15 minutes.

Questions

1. Six weeks ago the nurse and the midwife did a home visit to assess the home prior to determining if a home delivery would be appropriate for Marie. Make a list of the most essential things to be assessed in determining if Marie's home would be the best place for her birth.

2. List the equipment that the midwife and nurse bring to a home delivery.

3. Make a list of instructions the nurse or midwife needs to discuss with Marie, Eugene, and any persons who will attend the birth.

4. When the CPM and RN arrive at the house they find Marie to be 6 cm, 100% effaced, and at +1 station. Marie is walking around and breathing quickly through each contraction. What stage and phase of labor is Marie in?

5. The RN wants to assess the fetus. Describe how to use a Doppler to determine the fetal well-being at home. Include how to assess for periodic patterns.

6. The CPM and the RN begin to prepare the room for the delivery. Discuss the risk for infection in a home delivery as opposed to a hospital delivery.

7. Identify three preparations that will reduce the risk of infection for the baby and mother.

8. Marie's membranes break while she is walking around. The fluid is clear with a slight amount of blood streaking. What is the nurse's first concern and action at this time?

9. It is determined that the blood seen is just part of an increased show. What is the "bloody show?"

10. List five things the RN can suggest to the mother to cope with pain in labor.

11. How should the nurse monitor the contractions without an electronic monitor?

12. Marie delivers a healthy baby boy after one hour of pushing over an intact perineum. She chooses to deliver in the squatting position. What are the pros and cons of this position for delivery?

13. Marie is a primigravida. Why did the midwife choose not to do an episiotomy?

14. The midwife asks the nurse to examine the placenta. What should the nurse look for?

15. The placenta is delivered by "Shiny Schultz." What does this mean, and what are the implications if it had delivered by "Dirty Duncan?"

16. The baby nurses immediately after birth. The midwife puts the baby on Marie's abdomen (Actually both Marie and the midwife place the baby since the midwife encouraged Marie to assist in lifting the baby out of her.) The baby actually crawled to the breast and began to nurse on his own. Is this unusual? What factors in the hospital prevent babies from doing this?

17. After the birth and after the mother and baby are assessed, the nurse begins to clean the birth area. Can the nurse pour the bloody fluids down the drain? Is it safe to throw the placenta in the trash? If not, how should this be disposed of?

18. Describe the responsibilities of the nurse if a problem had been identified during the birthing process and it was determined necessary to transport the mother to the hospital for delivery.

Questions and Suggested Answers

1. Six weeks ago the nurse and the midwife did a home visit to assess the home prior to determining if a home delivery would be appropriate for Marie. Make a list of the most essential things to be assessed in determining if Marie's home would be the best place for her birth. There are several criteria that must be met for a home delivery to be conducted in the safest manner. The first of these is that there must be a ground floor area in the home for the birth. If the mother was to deliver in a room above the ground floor and there was a problem requiring a transport, it might be very hard to get her down a home staircase on a stretcher. Secondly, the home needs to be within 30 minutes of a backup hospital in case of the need for an emergency transport. Transportation must be available. An emergency care plan with instructions will have to be posted on the wall next to the phone, including the collaborating physician's name and phone number and the hospital phone number in case of need to transport. Running water and adequate environmental controls (heat in a cold winter and circulation in a warm summer) are necessary. Electricity or other source for adequate light and refrigeration for nutrition are desirable. A working toilet is necessary, and the home must be clean and free of pests and insects. Pets must be kept away from the birthing environment.

2. List the equipment that the midwife and nurse bring to a home delivery.
The equipment for a home birth includes: All appropriate paperwork for the chart and education of the mother postpartum; birth certificate or data form; reprints and reference materials for emergencies; stethoscope, sphygmomanometer, thermometer (for mother and for infant); urine chemstrips; nitrazine paper; sterile speculums; disposable premeasured (fleet) enema; catheter kit with straight catheter and Foley if needed; clean and sterile gloves; fetascope; Doppler with extra batteries; Doppler gel; olive oil; water soluble lubrication; iodine antiseptic solution; alcohol pads; bottle of betadyne; bottle of hydrogen peroxide; flashlight and batteries; bed pan and/or fracture pan; placenta bowl and large ziplock bags; amnihooks; hemostats; bandage scissors; instrument pan for sterilization; cold sterilization solution; slow cooker and tongs; birthing stool or chair; needle holder and pickups for suture; sterile 4″ × 4″ gauze; and vacuum tubes for cord blood collection. If the parents want to bank the infant's cord blood (for future use should the infant develop certain hematological or oncologic disorders), they will also need the special collection kit for this. The American Academy of Pediatrics currently does not support this practice; however, the choice is the parents' and they may request the midwives' assistance in this procedure.

For the baby: 3-ounce bulb syringe; tape measure; neonatal stethoscope; stockinet cap; cord scissors; cord clamp; portable baby scale; DeLee suction catheter with mucus trap; Res-Q-Vac or similar suction device; dextrostix; capped 4-ounce sterile D_5W baby bottles.

Medical drugs and supplies: herbal formulas and homeopathics including but not limited to black and blue cohosh, evening primrose oil; castor oil; caulophyllum; pulsatilla and moxa sticks; eye prophylaxis ointment; vitamin K; oxytocin (Pitocin) (10 IU vials for postpartum hemorrhage prevention or treatment); methylergonovine (Methergine) (0.2 mg vials and tablets); IV fluid D_5 in LR and LR; IV tubing; catheters tourniquet; antibiotics appropriate for client for GBS positive mothers; (D) immune globulin vaccination (RhoGAM) as needed; salts of ammonia or amyl nitrate (smelling salts); Lidocaine 1% or 2% in multidose vials; suture Vicril Rapide or chromic; needles; syringes; oxygen tank; tubing for oxygen and adult and infant masks; ambu bag for infant; laryngoscope with neonatal blade (extra batteries), check light; infant ET tube with stylet; infant airway; silk adhesive tape. Check all dates on sterile supplies and equipment.

The mother can be asked to supply the following: 25 chux under pads; diapers and clothes for the baby; several baby blankets and towels for immediately drying the baby; a plastic sheet to cover the mattress (may use a shower curtain); large sanitary pads; peri bottle; large plastic trash bags; ice packs (frozen moistened sanitary pads or gloves work well); heating pad; paper towels; flex straws; electrolyte replacement drinks (Gatorade or similar), protein foods and drinks for mother, and food for attendants and others at birth.

Also necessary are sterile bedding and equipment: 2 sets of sheets and pillow cases; two extra flat sheets; 4 soft bath towels; extra wash cloths for perineal compresses. The latter items may be sterilized by placing them in brown paper bags, folding the tops, and sealing with masking tape. Label the contents of each bag and bake in an oven at 250°F for 1 hour with a shallow pan of water on the bottom of the oven to prevent scorching. Do not let bags touch sides of the oven or each other. Keep bags closed until needed. Resterilize every fourteen days.

The parents may also want cameras, tape player with music, and so forth.

3. Make a list of instructions the nurse or midwife needs to discuss with Marie, Eugene, and any persons who will attend the birth. Marie should ask the people she wishes to be at the birth to also be present for the home visit. They should be people whom Marie is comfortable with and whom she desires to be there for her, not individuals who wish to be present for their own needs. Anyone present for the birth must be healthy, sober, and emotionally stable. The RN has less control over the environment at a home birth than she does in the hospital or birth center. For the mother, sometimes being able to limit the people she wishes to have present is just as important as including those she wants there. This meeting gives the midwife and nurse an opportunity to meet them, and for them to ask questions of the midwife and nurse. Parking should be discussed ahead of time. No cars should block the entrance of the home at the time of the labor and birth. This is to allow an ambulance to have easy and direct access to the main door if needed. If children are to be present, one adult per child needs to be at hand to attend to the child's needs. This adult needs to be ready to leave the birth with the child anytime the child indicates a need to leave or if the mother finds the child's presence too distracting. Children who are prepared for birth do very well; however, they cannot be expected to be on their best behavior when tension is high and labor is long.

4. When the RN and CPM arrive at the house they find Marie to be 6 cm, 100% effaced, and at +1 station. Marie is walking around and breathing quickly through each contraction. What stage and phase of labor is Marie in? Marie is in the active phase of the first stage, about to enter into transition.

5. The RN wants to assess the fetus. Describe how to use a Doppler to determine the fetal well-being at home. Include how to assess for periodic patterns. The nurse can use the Doppler to listen to the fetal heart tones for five seconds at a time then call out the numbers. The midwife or father then writes down these numbers, and they are recorded on a graph. This graph will give a visual of the baseline and long-term variability. There should be some variability easily identified on the chart, just as there is when an electronic monitor is continuously monitoring. Along with the fetal heart tones, the nurse needs to indicate when contractions are starting and stopping. If the heart rate decelerates and returns to the basline before the contraction ends, then the deceleration is probably a response to stimulation of the vagal nerve (pressure on the descending fetal head). This is a normal response. If the FHT decrease during a contraction and are still below the baseline at the end of the contraction, then the cause is probably related to hypoxia. This is called a late deceleration. When the FHT rise slightly then quickly fall below the baseline, then quickly rise above the baseline and then return to the baseline, the most likely cause is variable deceleration and is related to cord compression. A fetoscope may also be used for this. The midwife or nurse needs to listen to the heart through several contractions and continue to listen through the rest period between the contractions. Heart tones need to be listened to, assessed, and recorded at the same frequency as in the hospital.

6. The CPM and the RN begin to prepare the room for the delivery. Discuss the risk for infection in a home delivery as opposed to a hospital delivery. The best defense against infection is good hand washing. This is true for both in-hospital and out-of-hospital births. The risk for infection is greater in the hospital because the germs encountered are foreign and are a collection from many persons. In the home the mother is surrounded by an environment that she is accustomed to, both emotionally and bacteriologically. Her immune system has already developed immunity to the surrounding germs; and her immune system will function better when she is at rest, feels secure, and feels in control of her environment. In the last weeks of pregnancy the mother passes these immunities through the placenta to her baby. The limited number of care providers also greatly reduces her exposure to organisms. The family and caregivers are responsible for limiting attending persons at the birth and screening them for signs of illness.

7. Identify three preparations that will reduce the risk of infection for the baby and mother.

■ The number one intervention is hand washing. The nurse and midwife need to wash their hands when they arrive at the site and every time they care for the mother (and, later, the neonate).

■ Vaginal exams during active labor, and any time the membranes have ruptured, should be done infrequently and with aseptic techniques including sterile gloves. Hands should be washed both prior to putting on gloves and after taking them off. The nurse can also make sure that the doors are kept closed as much as possible to reduce air contamination.

■ The nurse can assess persons wishing to attend for signs of colds and other illnesses prior to their entering the birthing area.

8. Marie's membranes break while she is walking around. The fluid is clear with a slight amount of blood streaking. What is the nurse's first concern and action at this time? Any time a laboring woman's membranes break, the first nursing responsibility is to check the fetal heart tones to rule out prolapsed cord. This would be unlikely in this case since the baby is already at +1 station.

9. It is determined that the blood seen is just part of an increased show. What is the "bloody show?" Bloody show is a very wet mucous-like vaginal discharge with streaks of blood that accompanies active labor. It increases as the labor increases. It is normal. Heavy bleeding could indicate placenta abruption.

10. List five things the RN can suggest to the mother to cope with pain in labor. At home, the mother can take a shower at will and/or sit in her tub. The nurse can encourage her to use a birthing ball and offer her massage, including foot massages. The mother may wish to dance, sing, or pray. She is free to assume any position that she feels like. The home environment is free of intimidating strangers. The same woman who in the hospital is self-conscious about her behavior will feel free to sing (or moan) at the top of her voice, or dance with all of her heart at home. This ability to let go and move freely often is just what is needed to assist the baby's descent deeper into the birth canal. The mother instinctively changes to positions that feel better. Feeling better means moving the baby from areas of pressure, and doing these moves rocks the baby deeper into the birth canal. Mothers often assume hands-and-knees positions or squatting positions. These are excellent positions to increase comfort and move a baby along. Other helpful pain relievers are aromatherapy and using visualization.

11. How should the nurse monitor the contractions without an electronic monitor? Contractions need to be monitored just as frequently as in the hospital. By putting a hand on the fundus of the uterus the nurse can feel the beginning of the contractions, the intensity at the peak of the contractions, and when the uterus is relaxed. Intensity is described as strong when the fundus cannot be indented at the peak. Intensity is mild when the nurse or midwife can indent the fundus at the peak of a contraction. Between contractions the nurse feels to determine if complete relaxation occurs. All of these observations need to be assessed and recorded.

12. Marie delivers a healthy baby boy after one hour of pushing over an intact perineum. She chooses to deliver in the squatting position. What are

the pros and cons of this position for delivery? Women who are allowed to walk around in labor will often take a squatting position to push the baby out. This position opens the pelvic outlet as much as 2 cm more than a reclining position. It puts the baby into a position that directs him deeper into the birth canal and allows the mother to make use of gravity. The biggest disadvantage is that, if maintained for a long period of time, the mother's legs may tire and her perineum may swell, making it more prone to tearing. For this reason, she should squat when pushing and then stand, sit on a stool, sit at the edge of the bed, or lie back between contractions.

13. Marie is a primigravida. Why did the midwife choose not to do an episiotomy? There is usually no need to cut an episiotomy, even in a primigravida. When the midwife supports the perineum and or massages the perineum with hot compresses and oil, and the nurse coaches the mother to push gently, usually with small pushes between contractions, she can usually deliver the baby with an intact perineum. When a well-nourished mother is coached to work with the midwife to slowly deliver, and the midwife keeps the baby's head well flexed, she will seldom experience more than abrasions or a minor first-degree tear. The first-degree tears often do not even need suturing. Literature suggests that there is no benefit to the mother to do an episiotomy even when it appears that a laceration is imminent (Dannecker, Hillemanns, et al., 2004).

14. The midwife asks the nurse to inspect the placenta. What should the nurse look for? The nurse first needs to inspect the placenta to be certain that it is complete, then to observe for both membranes and to see if there are any vessels that look as if they could have been attached to extra lobes that might have been left behind. The nurse then estimates the size (normally the placenta is one-sixth of the weight of the baby). The nurse checks to see how healthy the placenta looks. Are there excessive calcium deposits or infracts that make it appear aged?

15. The placenta is delivered by "Shiny Schultz." What does this mean, and what are the implications if it had delivered by "Dirty Duncan?" A Shiny Schultz delivery means that the placenta comes out like an inverted umbrella with the shiny side out. This indicates a fundal attachment of the placenta. Duncan method is when the rough maternal side of the placenta comes out first, and usually means the placenta was located on the lower portion of the uterus. This area of the uterus does not contract after delivery as well as the fundus, and thus the postpartum bleeding is usually heavier with a Duncan delivery.

16. The baby nurses immediately after birth. The midwife puts the baby on Marie's abdomen. (Actually both Marie and the midwife place the baby since the midwife encouraged Marie to assist in lifting the baby out of her.)

The baby actually crawled to the breast and began to nurse on his own. Is this unusual? What factors in the hospital prevent babies from doing this? In a normal delivery with a normal baby, if the baby is not separated from his mother at all and the mother has not received drugs for the labor, the baby will be able to crawl to the breast, find the nipple, and begin to nurse. Studies on infant self-attachment for breastfeeding have shown that even a 20-minute separation between mother and baby after birth (as sometimes occurs when babies are taken from their mothers for initial assessment) decreases the likelihood of the baby finding the breast and latching on by his own efforts. When mothers receive pain medication in labor, the baby may not be able to crawl to the breast, latch on, or nurse.

17. After the birth and after the mother and baby are assessed, the nurse begins to clean the birth area. Can the nurse pour the bloody fluids down the drain? Is it safe to throw the placenta in the trash? If not, how should this be disposed of? If the home drainage system is a septic tank, the nurse will need to put these soiled materials into double red plastic bags, label them, and arrange for a special OSHA-approved agent to pick them up. If the drainage system is into a sewer system, it is safe to put them down the drain. Many midwives choose to put the placenta into a freezer bag and have it kept frozen for five days in case there is a reason for a pathology exam after the birth.

18. Describe the responsibilities of the nurse if a problem had been identified during the birthing process and it was determined necessary to transport the mother to the hospital for delivery. The nurse will follow the emergency care plan that was developed during the prenatal period. This includes calling 911, calling the backup physician and hospital to prepare them for receiving the mother, copying the chart, and assisting with oxygen or any other special management needs the mother has. The nurse and midwife will continue to monitor the mother and baby and prepare the family for the transport. They will reassure the family and give them direction. Either the midwife or the nurse will accompany the mother to the hospital and give a report to the medical team there.

References

Dannecker, C., Hillemanns, P., et al. (2004). Episiotomy and perineal tears presumed to be imminent: randomized controlled trial. *Acta Obstetricia et Gynecologica Scandinavica, 83*(4), 364–368

Sartore, A., De Seta, F., Maso, G., Pregazzi, R., Grimaldi, E., & Guaschine, S. (2004, April). The effects of mediolateral episiotomy on pelvic floor function after vaginal delivery. *Obstetrics & Gynecology, 103*(4), 669–673.

Varney, H., Kriebs, J., & Gegor, C. (2004). *Varney's midwifery* (4th ed.). Boston: Jones and Bartlett.

Catherine

AGE

14

SETTING

- Hospital labor and delivery unit

CULTURAL CONSIDERATIONS

- Black matriarchal culture

ETHNICITY

- Black American

PRE-EXISTING CONDITION

CO-EXISTING CONDITION/CURRENT PROBLEM

- Postdates; cord compression

COMMUNICATIONS

DISABILITY

SOCIOECONOMIC STATUS

SPIRITUAL/RELIGIOUS

PSYCHOSOCIAL

- Autonomy vs dependency

LEGAL

- Minor

ETHICAL

PRIORITIZATION

DELEGATION

PHARMACOLOGIC

- Epidural

ALTERNATIVE THERAPY

SIGNIFICANT HISTORY

- Primigravida

MODERATE

INTRAPARTUM

Level of difficulty: Moderate

Overview: This case requires critical thinking to assess cause-and-effect factors related to interventions and complications in labor and delivery. It requires assessment of factors related to postdate pregnancy.

Client Profile

Catherine is a 14-year-old, G1P0, single Black American teenager. She is admitted to the labor suite in active labor at 41 wga. Her pregnancy has been normal. She gained 28 pounds during the pregnancy. Her pelvis is gynecoid.

Case Study

Catherine's admission exam reveals the cervix 100% effaced, 6 cm dilatated, and the baby at −1 station; membranes are intact. Her contractions are every 5 to 6 minutes, moderate to strong, and lasting 1 minute. The FHT are 130s with good long-term variability (LTV) and occasional accelerations. Uterine relaxation is palpated between contractions. Catherine is tolerating the labor very well. At home she was walking around and dancing to relieve the contractions. She also finds that either singing or moaning with the contractions is a good distraction for her. She is in good spirits and pleased when she hears that she is already 6 cm. Her girlfriend, who also has a baby, is her coach; and they giggle between contractions. She brought her CD player to the hospital so that she could continue to play her music and dance. She has found that by rolling her hips with the dancing it gives her a lot of relief with the contraction pain. She has been having serious contractions for about seven hours. At home she ate a small amount of food and drank large amounts of juice, Gatorade, and water. Her pregnancy has been normal. Her admission vital signs are BP 128/68 (elevation in her systolic over her usual 110) pulse 84, respirations 20, and temperature 98.6.

Questions

1. Identify the coping mechanisms that Catherine is using and describe how they work.

2. Since her contractions are only moderate to strong and coming every 5 to 6 minutes, the obstetrician wants her to have Pitocin to increase their strength. Catherine refuses. Discuss the pros and cons of this order and the consequences of Catherine's refusal. She also refused the routine IV. Catherine's mother insists that she have the IV and she relents, crying.

3. Catherine's friend opens a lunch thermos and hands Catherine a cup of Gatorade to drink. The labor room standing orders are NPO in active labor. What is the rationale for the NPO order, and how might the nurse handle this situation?

4. Two hours after admission Catherine's contractions are 8 to 10 minutes apart. A vaginal exam (VE) indicates little change in her progress. What are the possible reasons for this?

5. The obstetrician decided to rupture her membranes during the vaginal exam to speed things along. The fluid is clear. She tells Catherine that she will have to have the Pitocin now because, if she does not resume labor and dilate, she may get an infection and endanger herself and the baby. The Pitocin is started. Catherine is in bed on an external monitor and beginning to feel very strong contractions. Twenty minutes after Pitocin is started the contractions are so strong that Catherine is crying and asking for something for pain. The FHTs are 130s with no accelerations and minimal long-term variability (LTV). A decision is made to insert a fetal scalp electrode to do internal monitoring. Contractions are every two minutes, lasting 90 seconds, and strong. Should the decision to rupture the membranes have been Catherine's?

6. How does it alter Catherine's labor?

7. What is the significance of the change in the FHT pattern?

8. What pain medication option might be available to Catherine? List the advantages and disadvantages of each.

9. Catherine's baby's heart rate decelerates to 100 bpm, then quickly rises to 150 bmp for 15 seconds, and then returns to the baseline of 130s. This happens three times in 10 minutes. What is the possible cause of this?

10. What nursing actions are necessary?

11. The doctor orders an amnioinfusion. What is this procedure, and why has he ordered it?

12. What are the nursing responsibilities when anmnioinfusin is ordered?

13. Catherine is given 800 mL IV of LR in preparation for an epidural. What is the rationale for this order?

14. Identify three nursing diagnoses that are appropriate for Catherine's care.

15. What the potential effects of the epidural on Catherine's baby?

Questions and Suggested Answers

1. Identify the coping mechanisms that Catherine is using and describe how they work. She is walking around and dancing to relieve the contractions. She also finds that either singing or moaning with the contractions is a good distraction for her. By moving freely and remaining upright, the baby is directed into the pelvis. This helps the baby to rotate and descend (Simpkin, 2002).

2. Since her contractions are only moderate to strong and coming every 5 to 6 minutes, the obstetrician wants her to have Pitocin to increase their strength. Catherine refuses. Discuss the pros and cons of this order and the consequences of Catherine's refusal. She also refused the routine IV. Catherine's mother insists that she have the IV and she relents, crying.

Advantage of Pitocin at this time: Since her contractions are less than every two minutes, the uterus could tolerate closer contraction and this might speed the labor.

Disadvantages of Pitocin at this time: The fetus is tolerating the labor very well now as evidenced by good baseline and accelerations without decelerations. Catherine is able to deal with the contractions well, and she is progressing very well. There is no need to hurry the process since her membranes are intact, mother and baby are doing well, and progress is occurring. Pitocin may increase the pain so that Catherine is unable to cope, forcing her to use pain medications. Stronger contractions could rob her of feelings of control, be detrimental to her self-esteem, and reduce her satisfaction of the experience of birth. Pitocin is a major cause of hypertonic contractions, which can rob the baby of needed oxygen and put the baby into distress. Pitocin also increases risk for rupture of the uterus, placenta abruption, birth trauma, and increased neonatal hyperbilirubinemia. In addition, although rare, the incidences of amniotic fluid emboli are increased with Pitocin usage.

The IV (needed for the Pitocin administration) is a painful invasive procedure. For the mother who is coping well with labor, this procedure can decrease her coping and increase her feelings of vulnerability. Having her mother insist that she take the IV undermines her sense of control. She is being treated as a child while having to function as a woman. Her crying at this demand is a reflection of this sense of vulnerability.

3. Catherine's friend opens a lunch thermos and hands Catherine a cup of Gatorade to drink. The labor room standing orders are NPO in active labor. What is the rationale for the NPO order, and how might the nurse handle this situation? Using IVs for hydration and keeping women NPO in labor is currently questioned as a standard of care for normal laboring women (Kubli, Scrutton, Seed, and O'Sullivan, 2002). This practice dates back to 1949 and currently is not supported by evidence-based studies. In the past, keeping a woman NPO in labor was considered safer care using the rationale that, if a woman were to need general anesthesia, it would be better if her stomach was empty to prevent aspiration (Mendleson's syndrome). This was based on studies that looked at the majority of women who received deep general anesthetics in the second stage. However, pregnant woman seldom have empty stomachs. Due to the influence of progesterone, the time it takes food to digest is much longer in the pregnant woman. Pregnant women also have the tendency to eat smaller, more frequent meals to reduce nausea. Therefore, care providers regard the pregnant woman as being at higher risk for aspiration due to the probability of food being in her stomach at any time. Even though the use of deep general anesthesia is no longer practiced, the very high rate of cesarean section has been used to continue this policy. However, general anesthesia is rarely used today, even for cesarean section, and when it is needed the technique for administration of anesthesia is improved. On the other hand, labor requires energy, and eating small amounts of nonfat food and drinking small amounts of energy-producing liquids can benefit the laboring woman. When IVs containing glucose are used to provide the laboring woman with energy and prevent dehydration, they may cause the infant to experience hypoglycemia. A fetus exposed to high levels of glucose (as when glucose-containing IVs are used) will respond by increasing her insulin levels. When the glucose IV is discontinued, it takes hours for the baby's insulin levels to adjust. The infant exhausts her glucose stores and the result is hypoglycemia shortly after birth. Maternal fluid overload and neonatal and maternal hyponatremia are also risks with IVs in labor.

4. Two hours after admission Catherine's contractions are 8 to 10 minutes apart. A VE indicates little change in her progress. What are the possible reasons for this? Catherine was progressing well when she could walk, move, and make her own decisions. It is not uncommon for contractions to slow for a period of time after hospital admission as the woman adjusts to the change in her surroundings. By providing support and encouraging Catherine to participate in her own decision making, the nurse can empower her to feel safe in this new environment.

5. The obstetrician decided to rupture her membranes during the vaginal exam to speed things along. The fluid is clear. She tells Catherine that she will have to have the Pitocin now because, if she does not resume labor and dilate, she may get an infection and endanger herself and the baby. The Pitocin is started. Catherine is in bed on an external monitor and beginning to feel very strong contractions. Twenty minutes after Pitocin is started the contractions are so strong that Catherine is crying and asking for something for pain. The FHTs are 130s with no accelerations and minimal long-term variability (LTV). A decision is made to insert a fetal scalp electrode to do internal monitoring. Contractions are every two minutes, lasting 90 seconds, and strong. Should the decision to rupture the membranes have been Catherine's? Any intervention or procedure should be explained to the mother, and she should be given the advantages, disadvantages, and consequences of such an action. Alternatives should also be explained. She should then have the right to accept or decline the intervention.

6. How does it alter Catherine's labor? By making the decision to rupture her membranes, the doctor made it necessary to use the Pitocin or risk infection from a prolonged labor.

7. What is the significance of the change in the FHT pattern? The baseline is rising; there is loss of accelerations and a decrease in LTV. These are all signs that the baby is being stressed; the most probable cause is the increased contractions resulting from the Pitocin.

8. What pain medication option might be available to Catherine? List the advantages and disadvantages of each.

	Narcotic	**Epidural**
Pros	**1.** Decreases perception of pain (takes the edge off) **2.** May allow rest between contractions	**1.** She will not feel pain **2.** Allows mother to rest
Cons	**1.** May cause respiratory depression of the newborn **2.** More difficult for the mother to maintain sense of control **3.** Interferes with natural endorphins **4.** May interfere with neonatal nursing	**1.** May cause maternal hypotension and decreased oxygen flow to fetus **2.** May increase neonatal jaundice **3.** May cause hyperthermia in the mother with resulting septic workup of baby **4.** Possibly interfere with mother's ability to direct pushing efforts **5.** Keeps mother non-mobile, which can interfere with fetal descent **6.** May interfere with the mother's ability to void, which will necessitate a Foley catheter, which in turn increases risk for bladder infections. **7.** Possibly increase risk for cesarean section **8.** Possibly cause chronic backaches and/or headaches **9.** May interfere with neonatal nursing

9. Catherine's baby's heart rate decelerates to 100 bpm, then quickly rises to 150 bmp for 15 seconds, and then returns to the baseline of 130s. This happens three times in 10 minutes. What is the possible cause of this? This describes variable decelerations, probably due to cord compression. Ruptured membranes, with an unengaged fetal head, increase the risks for cord compression and prolapsed cord.

10. What nursing actions are necessary? The nurse should do a vaginal exam to check for a prolapsed cord. Turning Catherine onto her side may relieve the pressure on the cord. If the contractions are closer than every two minutes and longer than 90 seconds, or if the resting tone is too high, then the Pitocin should be turned off. Increasing the amount of IV infusion (not containing the Pitocin) may also improve profusion to the fetus.

11. The doctor orders an amnioinfusion. What is this procedure, and why has he ordered it? Intact membranes allow the amniotic fluid to cushion the baby from the contractions; once the physician ruptured the membranes, more pressure was exerted directly on the fetus and cord. Amnioinfusion is a way of reversing this by temporarily adding fluid (normal saline or lactated ringers) to cushion the baby and cord. However, since the membranes have been ruptured this fluid will just drain out of the vagina so the effects are only short term. Amnioinfusion can also be used to dilute meconium stained fluid, thus reducing the risk from fetal aspiration. However, in this case the fluid is clear, so this does not apply. Initially 250 mL to 600 mL are infused into the uterus via dual intrauterine pressure catheters. One catheter is used to administer the fluid, and one is used to measure the uterine resting tone. This is done by an infusion pump or gravity flow at 10 to 15 mL/min.

12. What are the nursing responsibilities when anmnioinfusin is ordered? The fluid and all of the infusion equipment must be kept sterile. The fluid should also be warmed to room temperature and carefully monitored so that no more than 600 mL is infused without seeing fluid return. The nurse needs to observe for fluid return. Lack of adequate return and high uterine resting tone (above 20 to 25 mm Hg) are serious signs, and the nurse should stop the infusion. Other warning signs are maternal hypotension, shortness of breath, and tachycardia.

13. Catherine is given 800 mL IV of LR in preparation for an epidural. What is the rationale for this order? Epidural anesthesia reduces peripheral resistance, thus lowering blood pressure. This hypotension is one of the major dangers of epidural anesthesia in labor and may jeopardize the uterus to placenta circulation. Increased intravascular volume helps to maintain the mother's blood pressure when epidural anesthesia is used.

14. Identify three nursing diagnoses that are appropriate for Catherine's care.

- Potential for decreased fetal perfusion related to epidural anesthesia
- Altered urinary elimination related to epidural anesthesia
- Potential for delayed fetal descent related to bed rest

15. What are the potential effects of the epidural on Catherine's baby? Epidural anesthesia in labor has been associated with maternal fevers and increased neonatal jaundice. Both of these conditions require careful ruling out for infection and can result in additional testing and treatments that separate the mother and baby after birth.

References

American College of Obstetrics and Gynecology (ACOG). (2002). ACOG practice bulletin: Obstetric analgesia and anesthesia. *Obstetrics & Gynecology, 100*(1), 177–191.

Baumgarder, D. J., Muehl, P., Fisher, M., et al. (2003). Effect of epidural anesthesia on breast-feeding of healthy full-term newborns delivered vaginally. *Journal of the American Board of Family Practice, 16*(1), 7–13.

Blackburn, S. (2003). *Maternal, fetal, and neonatal physiology* (2nd ed.). Philadelphia: W. B. Saunders Co.

Himenick, S. (2003, March). Post ecstatic birth syndrome. *Vital Signs, 13*(5).

Kubli, M., Scrutton, M. J., Seed, P. T., & O'Sullivan, G. (2002). An evaluation of isotonic "sports drinks" during labor. *Anesthesia & Analgesia, 94*(2), 404–408.

Littleton, L., & Engebretson, J. C. (2002). *Maternal, neonatal, and women's health nursing.* Clifton Park, NY: Thomson Delmar Learning.

Mayberry, L. J., Wood, S. H., Strange, L. B., Lee, T., Heisler, D. R., & Nieslen-Smith, K., et al. (2000). Second-stage management: Promotion of evidence-based practice and a collaborative approach to patient care. Washington, DC: Association of Women's Health, Obstetric and Neonatal Nurses (AWHONN).

Rooks, J. P. (1999). Evidence-based practice and its application to childbirth care for low-risk women. *Journal of Nurse-Midwifery, 44*(4).

Simpkin, P., & O'Hara, M. (2002). Nonpharmacologic relief of pain during labor: Systematic reviews of five methods. *American Journal of Obstetrics and Gynecology, 186,* S127–S159.

Simpson, K. R., & Creehan, P. A. (2001). *AWHONN perinatal nursing* (2nd ed.). Philadelphia: Lippincott, Williams & Wilkins.

Peppie

AGE	**SPIRITUAL/RELIGIOUS**
24	■ Baptist
SETTING	**PSYCHOSOCIAL**
■ Hospital labor suite	
CULTURAL CONSIDERATIONS	**LEGAL**
■ Third-generation American; Northern European traditions	
ETHNICITY	**ETHICAL**
■ White American; Danish descent	
PRE-EXISTING CONDITION	**PRIORITIZATION**
CO-EXISTING CONDITION/CURRENT PROBLEM	**DELEGATION**
■ Postdate pregnancy; non-reactive NST; decreasing AFI	
COMMUNICATIONS	**PHARMACOLOGIC**
DISABILITY	**ALTERNATIVE THERAPY**
SOCIOECONOMIC STATUS	**SIGNIFICANT HISTORY**
■ Middle class	■ Multigravida

MODERATE

INTRAPARTUM

Level of difficulty: Moderate

Overview: Requires assessment of risks associated with postdate pregnancy and meconium-stained amniotic fluid. Requires understanding of fetal well-being testing used to evaluate the postdate fetus.

Client Profile

Peppie is a 24-year-old, MWF, G2P1001 who is admitted to the labor suite for induction at 42 weeks gestation. Until yesterday her biophysical profile was reassuring.

Case Study

This morning the non-stress test was non-reactive and the amniotic fluid index (AVI) was dropping. Peppie is unhappy about being induced, since she wanted a totally natural birth. Her mother, husband, doula, and sister are all with her. Peppie's last baby was born at home with a licensed midwife. The birth was long and hard, but Peppie describes it as "just beautiful." She had really hoped that this birth could be the same. Peppie plans to take her baby and leave the hospital six hours after the birth. Peppie's obstetrician artificially ruptures her membranes (AROM), and the fluid contains light to moderate meconium. On an external monitor the FHT are 110 to 120s with occasional accelerations and no decelerations.

Questions

1. What are the concerns when a pregnancy goes beyond 42 weeks?

2. What is the physiologic basis of the non-stress test, and what is the significance of a non-reactive test?

3. Peppie's amniotic fluid index is decreasing. Decreased amniotic fluid is associated with postmaturity. Why is this significant?

4. How safe is a planned home birth?

5. Peppie states that her last labor and birth were long and hard; however, she describes it as just beautiful. What are the most significant factors that influence how a mother feels about her birth experience?

6. How will induction affect Peppie's efforts at having a natural birth?

7. How can the nurse assist Peppie to achieve her own goals for this birth?

8. Discuss the pros and cons of early discharge.

9. Identify the teaching that needs to be emphasized if the mother and baby leave the hospital prior to 24 hours

10. What is the significance of the meconium in the amniotic fluid?

11. Is the initial FHT tracing reassuring or non-reassuring. Explain your answer.

Questions and Suggested Answers

1. What are the concerns when a pregnancy goes beyond 42 weeks? The placenta ages and the fetus grows larger, which may cause difficulty with birth. When the placenta becomes postmature the infant may actually lose weight, causing the head to be larger in proportion to the body (asymmetric); the fetus is less flexible, increasing risk of traumatic birth; there is increased risk of meconium aspiration as the amount of meconium increases in the fluid; and the total amount of amniotic fluid decreases, causing the meconium-stained fluid to be thicker.

2. What is the physiologic basis of the non-stress test, and what is the significance of a non-reactive test? When the fetus moves, he needs more oxygen. When the fetus is healthy, this need will cause a cardio–accelerator effect and increase the heart rate. If the fetus is compromised, this response will not occur, no acceleration of the heart rate will occur with fetal movement, and the test is considered to be non-reactive.

3. Peppie's amniotic fluid index is decreasing. Decreased amniotic fluid is associated with postmaturity. Why is this significant? This may indicate an aging placenta. In addition, the decreased fluid means more concentrated or thicker meconium and greater risk from aspiration.

4. How safe is a planned home birth? A planned home birth with licensed attendants is very safe. Infection rate is lower than in the hospital, and since planned home births do not utilize routine interventions, there are fewer complications. Studies that compared planned hospital birth with planned home birth found both equally safe and desirable for the low-risk woman and her infant (Olsen, 2004). The American College of Nurse Midwives (ACNM), MANA, and Lamaze International embrace out-of-hospital birth (birth center and homebirths) as safe birth options (Lamaze International Philosophy of Birth, 2003).

5. Peppie states that her last labor and birth were long and hard; however, she describes it as just beautiful. What are the most significant factors that influence how a mother feels about her birth experience? Ironically, the amount of pain a woman feels in her labor is not the most significant factor influencing her satisfaction with the birth experience. Repeated studies support the fact that when a woman feels that she has participated in the decision making, feels treated with kindness and respect, and feels empowered by her birth, her level of satisfaction is much higher than when she feels that everything is done to her, regardless of how much or how little pain she experiences (Nichols, 2000).

6. How will induction affect Peppie's efforts at having a natural birth? When contractions are induced, as opposed to natural labor, the labor results in more complications (Enkin, et al., 2000). Prostaglandins are first used to ripen the cervix, and this is followed by oxytocin (Pitocin) being administered through an IV on an infusion pump to stimulate contractions. Both may cause hard contractions. Inductions are usually managed in such a manner that the woman is brought very quickly to the point of hard active labor. Peppie is used to a long, slow, and gradual increase in her labor. When a woman is able to experience a naturally progressing labor, she gradually increases her tolerance to the strengthening contractions and her body responds by increasing its production of endorphins, nature's narcotic (Lamaze International, 2003). The induced, rapidly increasing labor will be much harder for her to tolerate and may require that she use medications that she did not wish to use. Also, monitoring contractions with Pitocin requires that the mother be on an electronic fetal monitor and have an IV. She will not be able to use some of the comfort measures that she used in her last labor. She may be restricted from walking, showering, or bathing, and assuming other positions that she had found helpful. Peppie may ask to have the Pitocin discontinued once active labor has been established (usually around 5 cm dilatation). At least one recent study suggests that continuing Pitocin after active labor has been established may be counterproductive by desensitizing uterine oxytocin receptors and that discontinuing it actually results in shorter labors (Daniel-Spiegel, et al., 2004). With the Pitocin discontinued she may be able to walk around.

7. How can the nurse assist Peppie to achieve her own goals for this birth? She can ask that the Pitocin not be advanced as quickly as is usual, allowing Peppie the opportunity to get used to the contractions, assist Peppie in changing positions, protect her privacy, advocate for her to have light food and liquids, encourage her to wear her own clothes, and generally support her and help to provide the comfort measures that the doula suggests. The nurse can also keep Peppie and her family informed of the progress.

8. Discuss the pros and cons of early discharge. The main problem with early discharge is that the family may not identify signs of problems with the baby or the mother. However, an educated mother and family and well-timed home visits can make early discharge very safe and desirable. With proper support, the home environment has many advantages for the mother and baby couple. Among these advantages are individualized care, family support, decreased exposure to infections, and maternal control of the environment, including total access to the infant.

9. Identify the teaching that needs to be emphasized if the mother and baby leave the hospital prior to 24 hours. Any mother leaving prior to or at 24 hours should have a planned home visit by a professional to assess the progress of the mother and baby and to offer teaching as needed. Teaching should include signs and symptoms of infection for both the mother and infant, signs of jaundice for the baby, signs of feeding and elimination problems in the baby, signs of excessive lochia, and DVT for the mother. Levels of activity need to be reviewed and adequate help at home needs to be established. Anticipatory guidance should be provided on infant feeding and care. The parents need to be able to recognize signs and symptoms of hyperbilirubinemia and know when to seek help. Trained and certified postpartum doulas can be very beneficial to the new mother.

10. What is the significance of the meconium in the amniotic fluid? Light meconium in amniotic fluid is not unusual when the infant is at, or near, term and may simply indicate a mature fetus. If the fetus is in a breech presentation, it is common for pressure on the presenting buttocks to cause meconium to be released into the amniotic fluid. In a small number of cases, meconium is released into the fluid when the infant is stressed. A brief episode of hypoxia causes the relaxation of the anal sphincter and release of meconium. Large amounts of meconium (thick or pea soup meconium), are either a sign of a very postmature infant or one that has experienced repeated episodes of stress. Once the meconium is present, the infant is at risk of meconium aspiration. Anything but light meconium requires careful suctioning of the infant just after the head is born. After the birth and before stimulation, the baby is suctioned deeply, and the cords are visualized and the baby suctioned to clear any meconium from the upper airway. This prevents meconium from the upper airway from being aspirated into the lungs when the baby begins to breathe. It is possible that the baby has aspirated meconium prior to the birth.

11. Is the initial FHT tracing reassuring or non-reassuring? It is reassuring. **Explain your answer.** Normal fetal baseline is 120 to 160 bpm. This baby is 110 to 120 bpm. However, since the baby is postmature the slightly lower baseline may be considered normal. Additionally, the presence of baseline variability and accelerations are both reassuring. This reflects a reactive baby who is able to increase her heart rate when there is a need for additional oxygen, such as when she moves. This is also the basis of the reactive non-stress test.

References

ACNM. Nurse midwives and home birth: Fact Sheet. (2004). http://www.acnm.org/prof/.

Blackburn, S. (2003). *Maternal, fetal, and neonatal physiology* (2nd ed.). Philadelphia: W. B. Saunders Co.

Daniel-Spiegel, E., Weiner Z., et al. (2004). For how long should oxytocin be continued during induction of labour? *BJOG: an International Journal of Obstetrics & Gynaecology, 111*(4), 331–334.

Enkin, M., Keirse, M., Neilson, J., Crowther, C., & Duley, L. E., et al. (2000). *A guide to an effective care in pregnancy and childbirth.* New York: Oxford University Press.

Himenick, S. (2003, March). Post ecstatic birth syndrome. *Vital Signs, 13*(5).

Jewell, O. O. (2004). Home versus hospital birth. *The Cochrane Library,* 3. Chichester, UK: John Wiley & Sons, Ltd.

Lamaze International. (2003). *Lamaze international position paper.* http://normalbirth.lamaze.org/About/PhilosophyofBirth.asp.

Littleton, L., & Engebretson, J. C. (2002). *Maternal, neonatal, and women's health nursing.* Clifton Park, NY: Thomson Delmar Learning.

Murphy, P. A., & Fullerton, J. (1998). Outcomes of intended home births in nurse-midwifery practice: a prospective descriptive study. *Obstetrics & Gynecology 92,* 461–470.

Nichols, F., & Humenick, S. (2000). *Childbirth education practice, research, and theory* (2nd ed.). Philadelphia: W. B. Saunders Co.

CASE STUDY 5

Lien

AGE

22

SETTING

- Hospital labor and delivery unit

CULTURAL CONSIDERATIONS

- Taiwanese traditions

ETHNICITY

- Asian

PRE-EXISTING CONDITION

CO-EXISTING CONDITION/CURRENT PROBLEM

- Acynclitism; prolonged second stage

COMMUNICATIONS

- Grandmother does not speak English

DISABILITY

SOCIOECONOMIC STATUS

SPIRITUAL/RELIGIOUS

- Buddhist

PSYCHOSOCIAL

- Conflicts in cultural practices; lonesome for her culture

LEGAL

ETHICAL

PRIORITIZATION

DELEGATION

PHARMACOLOGIC

ALTERNATIVE THERAPY

- Black cohosh

SIGNIFICANT HISTORY

- Primigravida

INTRAPARTUM

Level of difficulty: Moderate

Overview: This case requires application of culture sensitivity. It requires knowledge of the shape of the platypelloid pelvis and how it affects the mechanisms of labor.

Client Profile

Lien is a 22-year-old, G1P0, MAF at 38 wga. Her medical and surgical history are benign. She is a recent immigrant to the United States from Taiwan. She met her husband, who was working as an English teacher in Taiwan, three years ago. After two years of marriage they decided to come to the United States to settle and start a family. Although it was a mutual decision to move here, Lien is very lonesome for her family, her culture, and even her food. Her mother has come to be with her for the birth and postpartum. Her husband, an American, speaks Taiwanese very well, which makes it easier for everyone to get along. Her mother, Mia, is very traditional and a hard worker. She not only helps Lien get enough rest, but also cooks and cleans constantly. Lien's mother and her husband get along very well, but sometimes he is embarrassed by her traditional beliefs, especially when it comes to the pregnancy.

Case Study

It is 3 a.m., and Lien has been in labor for 18 hours. She is now 10 cm, 100% effaced, and −2 station. She has been pushing for 2½ hours. Lien is tired, and the nurse attempts to put cool wash cloths on her head to sooth her. Lien shakes her head and pushes the nurse's hand away. The contractions have gotten further apart and are now q 3 to 4 minutes and lasting 60 to 90 seconds but still strong. While the nurse is preparing to give Lien Pitocin to increase her contractions, Mia gently massages along the back of her heel in the indentation behind the tibia. Before the oxytocin (Pitocin) can be added to the IV, Lein's contractions are coming q 2 minutes and lasting 90 seconds. The external fetal monitor reveals a baseline of 140s with accelerations occurring between contractions. She has a few mild early decelerations with pushing. The baby is in the left occipital transverse (LOT) presentation during most of the pushing. Lien's mother steps in and helps her daughter into a hands-and-knees position for a few contractions. The baby moves to left occipital anterior (LOA) presentation and immediately descends to a +1 station. With the next two contractions the head is delivered. The shoulders are very tight but deliver with moderate traction. The baby needs some PPV and oxygen but the APGARS are 7 and 9.

After the birth, Mai asks her son-in-law (in Taiwanese) to ask for the placenta. Although the staff cannot understand what is being said, it is obvious that he is very uncomfortable with her request and at first just ignores her. Lien finally speaks up and tells the obstetrician that her mother would like to take the placenta home with her. Her husband rolls his eyes, and the obstetrician says that it is not possible because he has to send it to pathology for studies. Lien and Mia both look at each other with disappointment.

Questions

1. Prior to coming to the hospital for the birth Lien is given some herbs by her mother to help her in labor. These are traditional herbs used to nourish the uterus and help it to contract with more efficiency. Black cohosh is often used in Chinese medicine. How might the nurse find out about traditional herbs used by clients? How might these affect her labor in the hospital?

2. What is the most common pelvis for Asian women? How does it usually affect labor?

3. Why do you think Lien refused the cool wash cloths the nurse was attempting to put on her forehead for comfort?

4. Mia was a midwife in Taiwan for many years. Why did she have her daughter move to the hands-and-knees position? What did it accomplish?

5. Lien is in second stage for over two hours. What are the effects on the fetus when second stage is prolonged in an otherwise normal labor?

6. During the labor Mia gave Lien a drink of honey and herbs. How does this compare with the usual hospital policies on taking nourishment in active labor?

7. Assess the baby's heart rate during second stage.

8. What happened when Mia massaged Lien's ankles?

9. Why were the shoulders tight?

10. How can the nurse assist in the delivery of tight shoulders?

11. What are some of the traditions that Lien and Mia may practice during the postpartum that her husband may not understand?

12. Mia wanted the placenta to wash, dry, and make into a medicine for her daughter for postpartum. Discuss the husband's attitude and the response of the obstetrician. Do you feel that their actions were appropriate?

Questions and Suggested Answers

1. Prior to coming to the hospital for the birth Lien is given some herbs by her mother to help her in labor. These are traditional herbs used to nourish the uterus and help it to contract with more efficiency. Black cohosh is often used in Chinese medicine. How might the nurse find out about traditional herbs used by clients? There are several excellent books available on the use of herbs for medicinal purposes. The nurse can also directly and nonjudgmentally ask the mother what she has used. The woman will probably share this information if she feels she will not be criticized for using them. **How might these affect her labor in the hospital?** Black cohosh is a common herb used both by Chinese and European herbalists. It is an estrogen mimetic. Prior to labor and in early labor it is used to soften the cervix. It is used throughout the labor to regulate contractions. Black cohosh, however, may promote uterine bleeding, and thus its use near actual delivery time is discouraged.

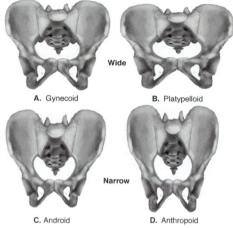

Wide

A. Gynecoid   **B.** Platypelloid

Narrow

C. Android   **D.** Anthropoid

Figure 2.1   *Female pelvis types. The platypelloid pelvis (B) is common in Asian women*

2. What is the most common pelvis for Asian women? How does it usually affect labor? Platypelloid is the most common pelvis found in Asian women (Figure 2.1). This type of pelvis tends to position the baby in the transverse position at the inlet with marked asynclitism. This can cause a delay at the inlet, which if not corrected may result in the need for cesarean section.

3. Why do you think Lien refused the cool wash cloths the nurse was attempting to put on her forehead for comfort? Cold and heat are important aspects to health in Chinese medicine. Lien and Mai would have viewed cold as interfering with the natural energy (chi) flow of body forces in labor, and therefore unacceptable.

4. Mia was a midwife in Taiwan for many years. Why did she have her daughter move to the hands-and-knees position? What did it accomplish? Mia used the weight of the baby's head and gravity to help the baby rotate from the LOT to LOA presentation in order to descend.

5. Lien is in second stage for over two hours. What are the effects on the fetus when second stage is prolonged in an otherwise normal labor? If the mother is able to rest between contractions and the resting tone between contractions is adequate, there are no harmful effects on the fetus in a prolonged second stage (Suzuki and Okudaira, 2004). However, the mother may be at increased risk for postpartum hemorrhage related to a fatigued uterus if contractions have been excessive.

6. During the labor Mia gave Lien a drink of honey and herbs. How does this compare with the usual hospital policies on taking nourishment in active labor? Although evidence-based practice does not support keeping a mother NPO in labor, many American hospitals still subscribe to the practice. As long as Lien drinks it slowly, it will provide hydration and energy for her labor. When women are left to their own accord in labor, they will naturally limit oral intake to liquids as the labor progresses. Oral intake of liquids provides not only hydration but also a sense of comfort for the laboring woman (Enkin, et al., 2000).

7. Assess the baby's heart rate during second stage. The pattern is very reassuring. The baseline was good, the accelerations are a reassuring sign, and the early deceleration indicates pressure on the fetal head (vagal nerve stimulation), which is a healthy sign, especially with pushing.

8. What happened when Mia massaged Lien's ankles? She stimulated a pressure point known to increase contractions. It worked, and the Pitocin was not needed.

9. Why were the shoulders tight? The platypelloid pelvis has short anterior–posterior diameter.

10. How can the nurse assist in the delivery of tight shoulders? The nurse can help position the mother in the McRobert's position, which brings the mother's bent legs far back, thus increasing the outlet diameters. Squatting will also open the pelvic outlet. If the shoulders are actually stuck (shoulder dystocia), the midwife or obstetrician may ask the nurse to push down just above the pubic bone (suprapubic pressure) to dislodge the shoulders. Another cause of tight shoulders is bed dystocia. If the mother is not far enough down on the bed to bring her hips over the end of the bed, the shoulders have a hard time rotating. This can be corrected by moving the mother down the bed so that her pelvis is beyond the end of the bed, or by using an inverted bedpan under her hips to allow space for the baby's shoulders to rotate.

11. What are some of the traditions that Lien and Mia may practice during the postpartum that her husband may not understand? Lien will not go out of the house or actually bathe (other than a sponge bath) for 30 days. She cannot wash her hair during this time. She will need to eat and drink a special mixture of herbs, which must be cooked fresh. These are meant to heal the uterus and promote breast milk production. Mia wanted the placenta to wash, dry, and make into a medicine for her daughter for postpartum. Dried placenta is thought to decrease postpartum depression.

12. Mia wanted the placenta to wash, dry, and make into a medicine for her daughter for postpartum. Discuss the husband's attitude and the response of the obstetrician. The husband was embarrassed by what he felt was a strange request. Most probably there had been some discussion about this prior to the birth. The obstetrician was misusing his authority to enforce his culture. There was no reason for the placenta to go to the lab. **Do you**

feel that their actions were appropriate? Unless there was some medical reason for sending the placenta to the lab, these were insensitive reactions on both their parts. The placenta does contain many hormones, and according to the Chinese culture it is considered an important part of the mother's recovery. The mother and daughter both felt disappointed. Their needs were not considered, and their culture was offended. It is possible that this could have been avoided if the family had felt comfortable enough to discuss their needs during the antepartum period.

References

Enkin, M., Keirse, M., Neilson, J., Crowther, C., & Duley, L. E., et al. (2000). *A guide to an effective care in pregnancy and childbirth.* New York: Oxford University Press.

Libster, M. (2002). *Delmar's integrative herb guide for nurses.* Clifton Park, NY: Thomson Delmar Learning.

Simpson, K. R, & Creehan P. A. (2001). *AWHONN perinatal nursing* (2nd ed.). Philadelphia: Lippincott, Williams & Wilkins.

Suzuki, S., & Okudaira, S. (2004, February). Influence of the duration of the second stage of labor on fetal pH levels and oxidative status in uncomplicated pregnancies. *Journal of Maternity Fetal Neonatal Medicine, 15*(2), 100–103.

CASE STUDY 6

Haiti

AGE

29

SETTING

- Hospital labor and delivery unit

CULTURAL CONSIDERATIONS

- Haitian immigrant

ETHNICITY

- Black; Haitian American

PRE-EXISTING CONDITION

CO-EXISTING CONDITION/CURRENT PROBLEM

- Unresolved grief; bereavement; delayed bonding

COMMUNICATIONS

DISABILITY

SOCIOECONOMIC STATUS

- Poverty; unsafe community

SPIRITUAL/RELIGIOUS

- Catholic and voodoo

PSYCHOSOCIAL

- Depression r/t recent loss

LEGAL

ETHICAL

PRIORITIZATION

- Needs to resolve grief prior to bonding with new baby

DELEGATION

PHARMACOLOGIC

ALTERNATIVE THERAPY

SIGNIFICANT HISTORY

- Multigravida; recent loss of 10-year-old son

INTRAPARTUM

Level of difficulty: Difficult

Overview: The case requires critical thinking for the student to assess the effects of grief on bonding. Some understanding of the Haitian culture is also needed.

DIFFICULT

Client Profile

Haiti is a 29-year-old, G2P1000, married Haitian female. Her first child, a 10-year-old boy, was killed two months ago while walking home from school. He was accidentally killed by a teenager who was drag racing, lost control of his car, and drove up on the sidewalk. Haiti's son was a quiet, straight "A" student who loved school, life, and most of all his mom and dad. He couldn't wait for his new little brother to be born. Haiti is now at 37 weeks gestation.

Case Study

At 2 a.m. Haiti is admitted in early labor to the unit. With each contraction she cries out in Creole "Oh God, why me? Why me, oh God?" and occasionally calls out her dead son's name. She appears to be in a trance. Her husband sits by her bedside, silently staring over her as if he doesn't even hear her. The labor progresses and a baby boy is born. The baby's APGARS are 9 and 9.

Questions

1. Describe the process of grieving. Give examples of this mother's behaviors that fit the grieving stages.

2. How does grieving the loss of the first child interfere with bonding to a new baby? Think of similar situations when this can cause a problem with maternal and paternal bonding.

3. How does grief affect the mother's ability to cope with contractions?

4. What could the nurse do during the labor to assist the mother?

5. When the baby is born, Haiti just turns her head away and cries even more. Explain the mother's behaviors.

6. What is the best way for the nurse to handle this situation?

7. What concerns for long-term problems does the nurse have?

8. What referrals can the nurse make for this family prior to discharge?

9. Haiti stays in the hospital for three days and is just starting to interact with her new son. Occasionally she calls him by his brother's name, and often she compares the two. Haiti had breastfed her older son and until recently had planned to breastfeed this baby. At the last minute she decides to bottle-feed. Why do you think she made that decision?

10. At three days the baby develops jaundice and the pediatrician decides it is best if the baby stays another day or two under the bili lights. Haiti begins to cry when she hears her baby is not being discharged with her. She cries out loud, "It's all my fault." How should the nurse respond?

Questions and Suggested Answers

1. Describe the process of grieving. According to Elisabeth Kübler-Ross (1969) the stages are:

1. Shock and denial
2. Disorganization and disorientation
3. Searching and yearning
4. Reorganization and reinvestment

Give examples of this mother's behaviors that fit the grieving stages.

1. *Shock and denial:* Avoiding looking at her new son after birth. Calling out her dead son's name.
2. *Disorganization and disorientation:* Difficulty in dealing with labor even at the earliest stages. Labor by itself is stressful and difficult. When a woman is grieving at this time, it can be even more difficult to maintain any organization to her coping; and pain becomes more painful, stress more stressful.
3. *Searching and yearning:* Calling out her son's name. Calling her newborn by his brother's name. She is having problems withdrawing the emotional investment she has in her dead son. This birth may cause her to recall her first son's birth, and she is finding herself preoccupied with his image and that past experience.
4. *Reorganization and reinvestment:* Her decision to bottle-feed is an example of her setting limits on her investment. Her distress at her baby not going home with her is a sign of her growing attachment for this baby or reinvestment in life.

2. How does grieving the loss of the first child interfere with bonding to a new baby? It is difficult to mourn one loss and develop an attachment to a new pregnancy or infant at the same time. **Think of similar situations when this can cause a problem with maternal and paternal bonding.** Similar situations may occur when one twin dies or there is a loss of a parent or partner during the pregnancy or right after the birth. Divorce or other termination of a strong relationship can also trigger these grief responses.

3. How does grief affect the mother's ability to cope with contractions? Grief brings extreme fatigue, and fatigue lowers the threshold for pain and coping. Her admittance during the early labor is an example of her not being able to tolerate even mild contractions at home. As a multipara, it would be expected that she not present until active labor.

4. What could the nurse do during the labor to assist the mother? The nurse needs to accept the mother's outcries and should not try to silence her. For some Haitian women, exaggerated movements and loud crying are cultural ways of expressing grief. For other Haitian women, complete silence and stoic behavior may serve the same purpose. The nurse needs to be readily available, even though it seems that the couple is not responding to their environment. The nurse needs to accept their behaviors and not try to make things better or fix things.

5. When the baby is born, Haiti just turns her head away and cries even more. Explain the mother's behaviors. Haiti may be afraid to make another close attachment, as she had with her son, knowing how much it would hurt if she lost this baby, too. She may also resent this baby taking the place of her other beloved son.

6. What is the best way for the nurse to handle this situation? Patience and listening are necessary at this time. The nurse needs to make time for the new parents and not force the baby on them. It is important that the baby is not taken to a nursery. Ideally, as soon as the mother indicates she is ready, the nurse should place the baby on the mother skin-to-skin. Holding the baby after birth causes a release of maternal oxytocin, which not only contracts the mother's uterus (aiding in the process of involution), but also causes the mother to feel calm and more responsive to her newborn. The nurse should also not force the baby into their arms until they reach for him, even if it takes time. If the mother or father wishes to compare this baby to their lost son, the nurse should listen, look at the pictures, and stay engaged in the conversation. The nurse should not try to distract the couple from this process.

7. What concerns for long-term problems does the nurse have? Haiti and her husband are still at a point in their bereavement where they are pre-occupied with the dead son. They may be more irritable and anger easily. It is difficult for them to maintain organized patterns of activities such as those needed to care for a newborn. The baby may be neglected or become an object of their anger. They may feel guilty for loving this baby and even feel that they are betraying their dead son by loving another. Haiti is also expressing feelings of guilt and transferring these to the newborn. (It's my fault—if I had done something differently he would not be hurting.) She may feel that if her son had been picked up after school and was not walking home that day, the accident would not have happened. They might expect this son to be perfect to make up for the loss of their other son.

8. What referrals can the nurse make for this family prior to discharge? The nurse can either search the Internet for support groups in her area or contact local hospitals for referrals. Examples from the Internet are: http://www.griefshare.org and http://griefnet.org/. The nurse may also find a local religious group or support person that the grieving couple can relate to. Support groups can be ongoing groups that provide a place for parents to go to talk, listen, and find support from one another. They can attend for as many sessions as they individually need. There are also support groups that provide regular structured support in the form of classes. These groups may have professionals involved and actually offer therapy, or they can mainly be run by other parents who have experienced losses. This mother will also need some help for the first few weeks at home. A postpartum doula would be a good referral.

9. Haiti stays in the hospital for three days and is just starting to interact with her new son. Occasionally, she calls him by his brother's name, and often she compares the two. Haiti breastfed her older son and until recently had planned to breastfeed this baby. At the last minute she decides to bottle-feed. Why do you think she made that decision? She may fear the closeness she had with her first son and not feel ready yet to make that attachment to this baby.

10. At three days the baby develops jaundice and the pediatrician decides it is best if the baby stays another day or two under the bili lights. Haiti begins to cry when she hears her baby is not being discharged with her. She cries out loud, "It's all my fault." How should the nurse respond? The nurse needs to use open-ended statements that allow Haiti to talk about her feelings. Just repeating back her statement as a question, "You're afraid it's all your fault?" may get Haiti to express her feelings. What is most important is that the nurse allow Haiti her feelings and not be judgmental of her. Haiti may be transferring guilt feelings about her son's death (If I had picked him up from school, etc.) onto the current situation with this baby. Guilt is a common response seen as a part of the grief work that a person progresses through after a loss. The nurse can also explain how jaundice is very normal for many babies. The nurse can talk to Haiti about ways that she can remain with her baby. Some hospitals have rooms where the mother may stay after her discharge if the baby is remaining in the hospital.

References

Anderson, G. C., Moore, E., Hepworth, J., & Bergmen, N. (2003). Early skin-to-skin contact for mothers and their healthy newborn infants. *The Cochrane Library,* 3. Oxford: Update Software.

Dunne, K. (2004, July). Grief and its manifestations. *Nurs Stand., 18*(45), 21–27, 45–51 & 52–53.

Greenspan, W. (2004). Why nurses need to understand the principles of bereavement theory. *Br J Nurs., 13*(10), 590–593.

Kübler-Ross, E. (1969). *On death and dying.* New York: Macmillan.

Littleton, L., & Engebretson, J. C. (2002). *Maternal, neonatal, and women's health nursing.* Clifton Park, NY: Thomson Delmar Learning.

Simpson, K. R., & Creehan, P. A. (2001). *AWHONN perinatal nursing* (2nd ed.). Philadelphia: Lippincott, Williams & Wilkins.

Minnie

AGE

29

SETTING

- Hospital

CULTURAL CONSIDERATIONS

- Modern medicalization culture

ETHNICITY

- Black American

PRE-EXISTING CONDITION

CO-EXISTING CONDITION/CURRENT PROBLEM

- Postpartum hemorrhage; fetal distress

COMMUNICATIONS

DISABILITY

SOCIOECONOMIC STATUS

- Middle class

SPIRITUAL/RELIGIOUS

PSYCHOSOCIAL

LEGAL

ETHICAL

PRIORITIZATION

- Desire to have husband present at birth vs risk from induction

DELEGATION

PHARMACOLOGIC

- Dinoprostone (Cervidil); oxytocin (Pitocin); epidural

ALTERNATIVE THERAPY

SIGNIFICANT HISTORY

- Multigravida

DIFFICULT

INTRAPARTUM

Level of difficulty: Difficult

Overview: This case presents multiple complications. The nurse in this scenario needs to identify cause and effect when assessing long- and short-term pros and cons of various interventions in labor. She is asked to compare and contrast procedures. She needs background knowledge of medications used to induce labor and to know how to assess fetal heart rate.

Client Profile

Minnie is a 29-year-old, G2P1001, MBF, who is having her labor induced at 38 wga. Her last delivery was induced and she received an epidural anesthesia one year ago. She had a seven-pound baby boy after birth, and he was kept in the NICU for 24 hours under observation and for a septic workup because she had developed a fever during the delivery. The antibiotics were discontinued after 48 hours when all cultures were negative. He did have elevated bilirubin and required three days under the bili light. At four days the baby developed thrush, and Minnie also got the thrush on her nipples. Although she had planned to breastfeed, all of the unanticipated problems and delays in being able to keep the baby with her at the bedside and the sore nipples with thrush discouraged her, and by day seven she decided to bottle-feed. She is anxious about this delivery and has been dreading it since she got pregnant.

Case Study

She was admitted last night at 7 p.m. for dinoprostone insertion (Cervidil) to ripen the cervix in anticipation of a Pitocin induction this morning. Minnie requested the induction (with the encouragement of her physician) because her husband would be out of town starting in two weeks when she will be 40 weeks. Her admission Bishop score was 2 (cervix is soft and midline).

Questions

1. Minnie is having an elective induction (no medical indication). What are the pros and cons of this decision?

2. What does her Bishop score mean?

3. In her first delivery infection was ruled out as a cause of maternal fever; what else might have been the cause?

4. What are the causes of elevated bilirubin in neonates? What was the most likely cause of Minnie's first baby's jaundice?

5. What is the most likely reason why the baby developed thrush?

6. What other sources are there for this infection?

7. Do you think Minnie will breastfeed this time? How might the nurse encourage it?

8. At 10 a.m. Pitocin is started. The obstetrician ruptures her membranes, and the fluid is clear. Minnie's cervix is soft, midline, 30% effaced, and fingertip dilated. The baby is −2 station. By 10:30 a.m. she is contracting regularly every three minutes for one minute and having strong contractions. The FHT are in the 130s with occasional accelerations. By 11:30 a.m. her contractions are every two minutes, 60 to 90 seconds in length, and strong. An internal scalp electrode is placed and indicates minimal short-term variability. There are no more accelerations. There are no decelerations. FHTs baseline is in the 140s. Minnie requests an epidural. She receives a bolus of 1000 mL LR IV, and the epidural is given. Describe the changes that are occurring in the FHT patterns and give possible reasons for them.

9. At 3 p.m. Minnie is 5 cm, 100% effaced, and the baby is at −1 station. Fluid remains clear and non-odorous. Minnie is sleeping. FHT are in the 140s with minimal baseline variability, no accelerations, and occasional variable decelerations with quick return to baseline. A Foley catheter has been inserted into Minnie's bladder and 700 mL clear pale urine is obtained. When should the Pitocin be increased? When should it be decreased?

10. How does a full bladder impact on labor?

11. What is the significance of the increasing FHT baseline?

12. What are the possible reasons for the variable decelerations?

13. What nursing actions are needed?

14. After two more hours Minnie is checked and found to be complete complete (10 cm dilatated and 100% effaced). She has difficulty pushing. A mediolateral episiotomy is performed, and the baby's head is delivered with the assistance of a vacuum extractor (Figure 2.2). The baby initially needed positive pressure ventilation (PPV) with 100% oxygen. His APGARS were 5 and 7. The episiotomy

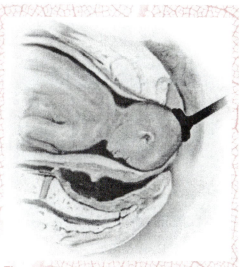

Figure 2.2 *Vacuum-assisted birth*

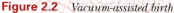

extends to a fourth-degree laceration. Her estimated blood loss (EBL) is 700 mL. What possible problems can you predict with Minnie's postpartum?

15. Can you anticipate any problems for this baby?

16. Using critical thinking to compare and contrast interventions, risks, and benefits, can you visualize how this labor and delivery might have been handled in a different manner with a different outcome?

Questions and Suggested Answers

1. Minnie is having an elective induction (no medical indication). What are the pros and cons of this decision? The only advantage to this decision is that the mother can schedule her delivery, in this case when her husband is going to be in town. Dangers include delivering a preterm baby, failed induction with cesarean section, prolonged induction with maternal exhaustion, prolonged use of Pitocin, which may increase neonatal jaundice and put mother at risk for water intoxication as well as increased risk of postpartum hemorrhage, and increased possibility for infection (Kramer, et al., 2000). There is also a greater possibility of the need for increased pain relief, including epidurals, which can cause hypotension and maternal fever (Lieberman and O'Donoghue, 2002).

2. What does her Bishop score mean? This is a method of determining the likelihood of the cervix being inducible. Prostaglandins are used to increase the possibility that an induction with oxytocin (Pitocin) will be effective. Minnie has a low Bishop score initially, which means there is a low chance of successful induction unless the prostaglandins improve the score. That is why she was admitted the night before. If the Bishop score did not improve, she could have received another dose of prostaglandins. Bishop score is used to provide an objective assessment of how probable it is that an induction will produce an effective labor. It evaluates how soft the cervix is, the position of the cervix, if it is effaced, if it is dilatated, and what station the baby is at.

3. In her first delivery infection was ruled out as a cause of maternal fever; what else might have been the cause? The most likely cause was the maternal epidural. Dehydration and infections must always be ruled out.

4. What are the causes of elevated bilirubin in neonates? Physiologic jaundice is the most common cause. Dehydration can also increase bilirubin levels. Maternal epidurals have been associated with increased jaundice in the baby. **What was the most likely cause of Minnie's first baby's jaundice?** Minnie had both an epidural and Pitocin induction. These may have added to the normal physiologic jaundice, bringing levels up so that the pediatrician felt that phototherapy was necessary. In addition, if the baby was not able to stay with Minnie at the bedside, she might not have been nursing frequently enough and this too could add to dehydration. Although breast milk has been known to increase benign jaundice, it was too early for this to be a reason in her case. If the baby had had an infection, then the infection might also have contributed to higher bilirubin levels since infection is often accompanied by red blood cell lysis.

5. What is the most likely reason why the baby developed thrush? The antibiotics are the most likely cause for this. Another source is cross-contamination from caregivers' hands.

6. What other sources are there for this infection? If Minnie had had a fungal vaginal infection at the time of birth, this might also cause thrush in the neonate.

7. Do you think Minnie will breastfeed this time? This is unlikely. Minnie had a negative experience last time, and it is probable that the baby will also have increased bilirubin (epidural, Pitocin, and possible increased RBC breakdown from minor trauma during the birth resulting from the vacuum extraction and tight shoulders). In addition, this time Minnie will be recovering from an increased blood loss (making her more tired) and a painful perineum from the episiotomy and fourth-degree tear. **How might the nurse encourage it?** The nurse can encourage her to breastfeed by having a lactation consultant visit her soon after delivery, encourage her to breastfeed at the delivery, and encourage a family member to stay with her, thereby allowing her to have the baby with her at all times. She may also suggest a postpartum doula to help her at home.

8. At 10 a.m. Pitocin is started. The obstetrician ruptures her membranes, and the fluid is clear. Minnie's cervix is soft, midline, 30% effaced, and fingertip dilated. The baby is −2 station. By 10:30 a.m. she is contracting regularly every three minutes for one minute and having strong contractions. The FHT are 130s with occasional accelerations. By 11:30 a.m. her contractions are every two minutes, 60 to 90 seconds in length, and strong. An internal scalp electrode is placed and indicates minimal short-term variability. There are no more accelerations. There are no decelerations. FHTs baseline is in the 140s. Minnie requests an epidural. She receives a bolus of 1000 cc LR IV, and the epidural is given. Describe the changes that are occurring in the FHT patterns and give possible reasons for them. As the contractions become stronger, closer, and longer, the baby begins to show sign of stress. Loss of accelerations and decreased variability may be due to fetal sleep; however, since they do not return within 80 minutes, these are more likely to be early signs of stress.

9. At 3 p.m. Minnie is 5 cm, 100% effaced, and the baby is at −1 station. Fluid remains clear and non-odorous. Minnie is sleeping. FHT are in the 140s with minimal baseline variability, no accelerations, and occasional variable decelerations with quick return to baseline. A Foley catheter has been inserted into Minnie's bladder and 700 mL clear pale urine is obtained. When should the Pitocin be increased? The Pitocin should not be increased since the contraction pattern has reached the most intense that is desirable, and any increase would cause hyperstimulation and increased fetal stress. Effects on the uterus from hyperstimulation include possible placenta abruption, uterine rupture, and postpartum hemorrhage (PPH) due to fatigue and the resulting atony. The baby could show increasing signs of fetal distress as oxygen delivery is interfered with when the uterus does not have adequate time to relax between contractions. **When should it be decreased?** The Pitocin needs to be discontinued at any sign of fetal distress. Newer studies also recommend stopping it when the mother reaches 5 cm. In a recent article in the *British Journal of Obstetrics and Gynecology*, Daniel-Spiegel suggests that there is no benefit to continuing oxytocin infusion after the onset of active labor. The article also discusses previous research that examines the effect of continuous oxytocin infusion on the number and behavior of oxytocin receptors, which suggests that there may be a point at which administering more oxytocin begins to desensitize uterine receptors, which in turn may have an opposite effect on the progress of labor when labor induction is undertaken. These authors suggest that continuing oxytocin infusion beyond the onset of active labor may interfere with labor progress (Daniel-Spiegel, et al., 2004).

10. How does a full bladder impact on labor? Descent of the baby may be impaired by a full bladder. A full bladder at delivery can also contribute to a severe hemorrhage immediately after the delivery of the placenta because it can push the uterus to the side, thus preventing the uterus from contracting. Finally, trauma to the bladder can occur if the delivery is forced. Women who have full bladders in labor and do not have epidurals also experience increased pain.

11. What is the significance of the increasing FHT baseline. There is an increase in the FHT baseline. This may be an early sign of maternal infection. The nurse should check the maternal temperature more frequently.

12. What are the possible reasons for the variable decelerations? This is another sign of fetal stress. The variable decelerations may have been caused from cord compression as occurs when the membranes are ruptured. This baby was not engaged, increasing the possibility of cord compression and prolapse. The quick return to baseline is a good sign.

13. What nursing actions are needed? Nursing actions include changing the mother's position and closely monitoring for changes in the variable deceleration patterns that may necessitate giving the mother oxygen and turning off the Pitocin. Increasing IV fluids without Pitocin sometimes also helps to reduce fetal stress.

14. After two more hours Minnie is checked and found to be complete complete (10 cm dilatated and 100% effaced). She has difficulty pushing. A mediolateral episiotomy is performed, and the baby's head is delivered with the assistance of a vacuum extractor. The baby initially needed positive pressure ventilation (PPV) with 100% oxygen. His APGARS were 5 and 7. The episiotomy extends to a fourth-degree laceration. Her estimated blood loss (EBL) is 700 mL. What possible problems can you predict with Minnie's postpartum?

- Minnie has experienced a PPH and a fourth-degree laceration. Both increase her risk for infection.
- She may also be fatigued from the blood loss, although this may be minimal if her prenatal H&H was high enough.
- She is at increased risk of UTI due to the Foley catheter and may experience problems with voiding initially after the Foley is removed.
- She may have problems with fecal incontinence from the fourth-degree laceration.

- She will have aching in her legs and lower back from the McRobert's position.
- The fourth-degree laceration will cause pain.
- She may experience constipation related to narcotic pain medications and fear of having a BM.
- She may experience chronic backache related to the epidural anesthesia and/or position in labor.
- She is more likely to experience diaphoresis related to the increased IV fluids she was given in labor.

15. Can you anticipate any problems for this baby? This baby is at risk for increased jaundice related to Pitocin and epidural use as well as bruising resulting from the vacuum extractor. The baby may need a septic workup if the mother developed a fever in labor. Because of the stressful delivery, the baby may become hypoglycemic and initially have problems maintaining her temperature.

16. Using critical thinking to compare and contrast interventions, risks, and benefits, can you visualize how this labor and delivery might have been handled in a different manner with a different outcome?

Current Case	Problem	Alternative Actions
Non-medical induction	Need for AROM, prostaglandin, and Pitocin-stressed baby, possible cause of increased neonatal bilirubin	Wait until labor starts
Epidural	Vacuum extraction leading to increased bruising and increased bilirubin for the baby. Need for sepsis workup on baby r/t maternal fever	Support and natural labor and delivery without medications interfering with fetal descent and maternal pushing efforts
	For the mother: Increased laceration and blood loss	

Summary

Intervention effects on mother: Inductions for non-medical reasons lead to use of Pitocin prior to natural cervical ripening, often leading to need for epidural, which decreases maternal ability to change positions and causes delays in fetal rotation and descent during first stage. Epidurals also lead to use of Foley catheters. In second stage there is an inability to change positions for pushing, which further leads to need for vacuum extractor or forceps. The vacuum extractor (or forceps) in turn lead to the need for a large mediolateral (ML) episiotomy, which may cause fourth-degree lacerations (lacerations through the rectal sphincter and into the rectal mucosa). These lacerations cause extensive blood loss, greater postpartum pain, increased potential for infection, and possible long-term bowel incontinence.

Intervention effects on infant: AROM prior to engagement may lead to cord compression and increased stress on infant from lack of cushioning. Pitocin-induced strong contractions lead to stress on infant. Fetal stress may have contributed to infant's poor coping with stress of second stage, requiring increased resuscitation efforts.

Epidural anesthesia reduces the position options available to the mother and reduces her ability to directly push the baby out. This increases the need for vacuum extraction or forceps (Lamaze International, 2003). Infant will probably have increased jaundice due to trauma from vacuum extractor. If mother developed a fever (common response to the epidural anesthesia), the baby would have required a septic workup, which usually results in longer mother–baby separation, formula supplementation, and decreased breastfeeding.

References

Daniel-Spiegel, E., Weiner Z., et al. (2004). For how long should oxytocin be continued during induction of labour? *BJOG: an International Journal of Obstetrics & Gynaecology, 111*(4), 331–334.

Kramer, M. S., Demissie, K., Platt, R. W., Sauve, R., & Liston, R. (2000). The contribution of mild and moderate preterm birth to infant mortality. *JAMA, 284*(7), 843–849.

Lamaze International (2003). *Lamaze international position paper.* http://www.lamaze.org.

Lieberman E., & O'Donoghue, C. (2002). Unintended effect of epidural anesthesia during labor: a systemic review. *American Journal of Obstetrics and Gynecology, 186*(5), S31–S68.

Littleton, L., & Engebretson, J. C. (2002). *Maternal, neonatal, and women's health nursing.* Clifton Park, NY: Thomson Delmar Learning.

Simpson, K. R, & Creehan, P. A. *AWHONN perinatal nursing* (2nd ed.). Philadelphia: Lippincott, Williams & Wilkins.

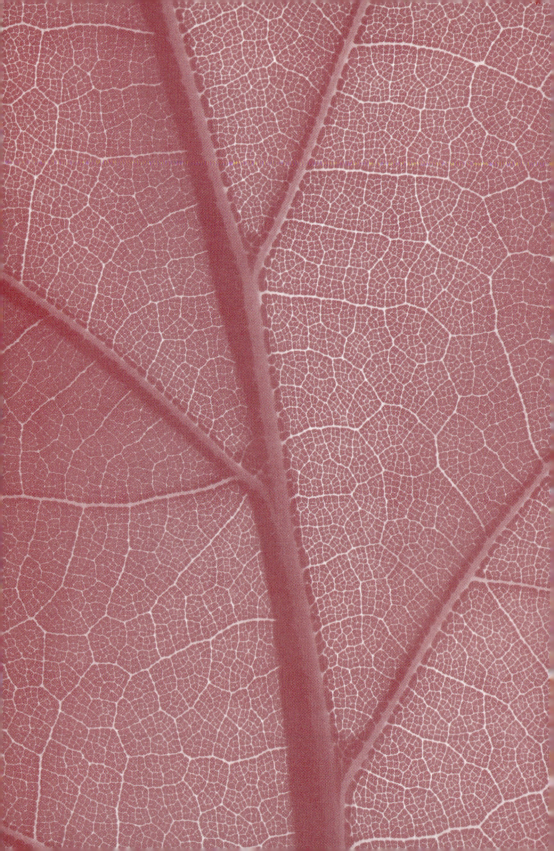

PART THREE

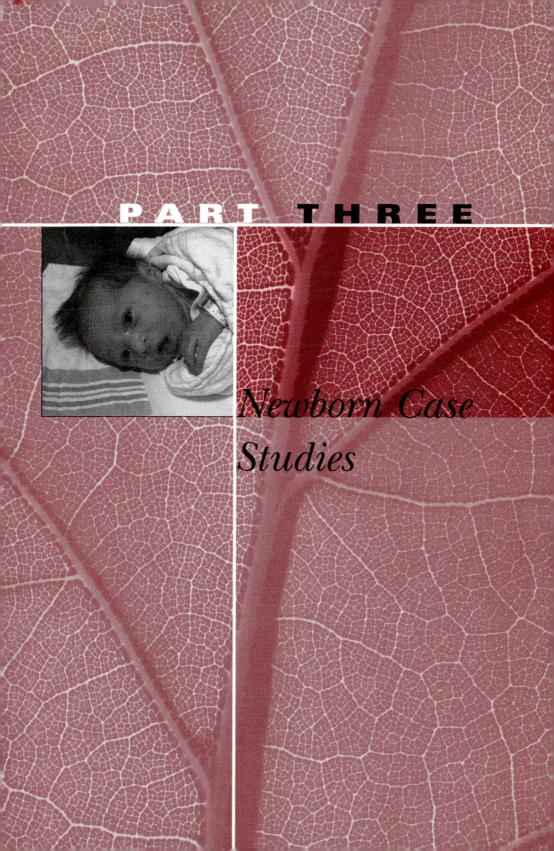

Newborn Case Studies

CASE STUDY 1

Baby Brooks

AGE

28 hours

SETTING

- Hospital nursery

CULTURAL CONSIDERATIONS

- White urban American values

ETHNICITY

- White American

PRE-EXISTING CONDITION

CO-EXISTING CONDITION/CURRENT PROBLEM

COMMUNICATIONS

DISABILITY

SOCIOECONOMIC STATUS

SPIRITUAL/RELIGIOUS

PSYCHOSOCIAL

LEGAL

ETHICAL

PRIORITIZATION

DELEGATION

PHARMACOLOGIC

ALTERNATIVE THERAPY

SIGNIFICANT HISTORY

- Delivered by NSVD

NEWBORN

Level of difficulty: Easy

Overview: Requires knowledge regarding male circumcision, including cultural preferences and care of infants both circumcised and uncircumcised.

Client Profile

Baby Brooks is a 28-hour-old boy. He was born full term with APGARS of 8 and 9 via a NSVD. He is being breastfed. He is active and alert.

Case Study

Baby Brooks's mother seems agitated when the nurse comes to check her at the beginning of the afternoon shift. When the nurse asks her what seems to be the problem, she states, "My husband wants to have our son circumcised and I don't want to. What do you think we should do?"

Questions

1. List the most common reasons that male circumcision is done.

2. What is the incidence of male circumcision in the United States today?

3. In which religions is circumcision considered a religious rite?

4. In which religions is circumcision absent?

5. Define the following terms:
Phimosis
Balanoposthitis
Paraphimosis

6. List three complications associated with circumcision.

7. Outline the most recent Academy of Pediatrics position statement on routine male circumcision.

8. Describe the pain relief measures that can be used when male circumcision is performed.

9. Describe the nursing care of the infant post-circumcision.

10. Outline the instructions given to parents of an uncircumcised male infant.

Questions and Suggested Answers

1. List the most common reasons that male circumcision is done. The most common reasons given for male circumcision are religious and cultural. There may also be medical concerns from questionable studies related to prevention of infection and decreasing risk of cancer.

2. What is the incidence of male circumcision in the United States today? At least 61% of males in the United States are circumcised. That figure is probably under-reported.

3. In which religions is circumcision considered a religious rite? Both Judaism and the Muslim faith circumcise males as a religious rite.

4. In which religions is circumcision absent? Hindu-Buddhist and Confucian religions do not advocate circumcision as a part of their faith. The Christian church has no specific doctrine on circumcision.

5. Define the following terms:

Phimosis: Narrowing of foreskin that prevents retraction

Balanoposthitis: Inflammation of the glans penis and mucus membranes; it is usually mild and self-limiting

Paraphimosis: A retracted, tight foreskin that cannot be replaced

6. List three complications associated with circumcision. Complications that can occur as a result of circumcision are bleeding, local infection, sepsis, amputation, nectrotizing fasciitis, meningitis, and death.

7. Outline the most recent Academy of Pediatrics position statement on routine male circumcision. There are two main points in the 1999 position statement. The first of these states that although not sufficient to recommend routine circumcision, circumcision does protect from urinary tract infections, penile cancer, and various sexually transmitted infections. Secondly, it takes a position that circumcision is painful, and pain relief should be used.

8. Describe the pain relief measures that can be used when male circumcision is performed. Dorsal penile nerve block may be used for infant circumcision. Note that lidocaine-prilocaine cream (EMLA) is not recommended for use in infants under 1 month.

9. Describe the nursing care of the infant post-circumcision. Carefully remove and apply diaper to avoid rubbing at the site. Check the site for bleeding every 30 minutes for the first two hours and then every two hours for the remainder of the first 24 hours. Observe for voiding. Following a circumcision, the infant who voids less than six times in 24 hours needs to be assessed. If a dressing has been applied, it needs to be removed, the penis assessed, and the dressing changed at least three times in the first 24 hours. Acetaminophen drops can be given for pain. Keep the glans clean with plain water. Do not attempt to remove the yellow exudates that form on the glans on the second day; this is part of the healing process. K-Y Jelly or ointment may be used under the dressing if a plastic ring was not used for the circumcision. Do not use these if a ring was applied since they may cause the ring to fall off too early. Report signs of infection.

10. Outline the instructions given to parents of an uncircumcised male infant. Do not forcibly retract the foreskin. This will occur naturally as the child grows. Clean with plain water.

References

American Academy of Pediatrics. (1998). *American academy of pediatrics circumcision policy statement.* http://www.aap.org/.

Littleton, L., & Engebretson, J. C. (2002). *Maternal, neonatal, and women's health nursing.* Clifton Park, NY: Thomson Delmar Learning.

Updegrove, K. (2001). An evidence-based approach to male circumcision: What do we know?. *Journal of Midwifery & Women's Health, 46*(6).

CASE STUDY 2

Baby Taber

AGE

48 hours

SETTING

- Hospital postpartum unit

CULTURAL CONSIDERATIONS

ETHNICITY

- Hispanic American

PRE-EXISTING CONDITION

- Maternal diabetes

CO-EXISTING CONDITION/CURRENT PROBLEM

- Infant of diabetic mother; engorgement

COMMUNICATIONS

DISABILITY

SOCIOECONOMIC STATUS

SPIRITUAL/RELIGIOUS

PSYCHOSOCIAL

LEGAL

ETHICAL

PRIORITIZATION

DELEGATION

PHARMACOLOGIC

- Stadol

ALTERNATIVE THERAPY

SIGNIFICANT HISTORY

- Delivered by cesarean section

NEWBORN

Level of difficulty: Moderate

Overview: Requires understanding of the effects of maternal diabetes on the newborn. Requires knowledge concerning benefits and process of breastfeeding.

Client Profile

Baby Taber is a 48-hour-old, Hispanic American newborn. He was born via cesarean section for breech presentation at 38⅔ weeks gestation. The prenatal course was normal. His mother gained 28 pounds during the pregnancy. He is the first baby in the family. His birth weight was 9 pounds 2 ounces. He is being breastfed approximately every two hours around the clock, except last night when he was given a bottle of formula in the nursery.

Case Study

Baby Taber's mother is attempting to breastfeed her baby, and the baby is having problems latching on. The nurse notes that her breasts are engorged. The mother is crying when the nurse arrives in the room; she has many questions concerning her baby. When she was reviewing her baby's chart she noticed that he had been given some glucose water shortly after his birth. She asks the nurse why this was done. She had specifically asked that he not be given any bottles. She wants to know why the baby, who was nursing so well yesterday, suddenly cannot seem to latch on this morning. She also noticed that the baby's stools are very smelly when they were not yesterday. She questions the nurse about the baby's eyes, which tend to cross once in awhile. She is also concerned that the baby's "soft" spot on the top of his head seems to bulge when he is crying or sucking hard. The nurse notes that the baby is slightly jaundiced.

Questions

1. Baby Taber is the infant of a diabetic mother. What are the signs of hypoglycemia? How is the baby tested for hypoglycemia? What is the normal range blood sugar for a newborn right after birth?

2. Explain to the mother why the baby was given glucose water shortly after birth.

3. What other problems may occur in the infant of a diabetic mother (IDM)?

4. The mother distinctly told the staff that she only wanted the baby to get breast milk. The night nurse working in the nursery decided that, since the mother had had a cesarean section and had been nursing all day, she was tired, and that giving the baby one bottle of formula would give her a rest and would do no harm. Discuss this nursing decision and the validity of her conclusions.

5. Why is the baby now having problems latching on?

6. Discuss normal newborn stool patterns, including odor and consistency. What is the significance of a "smelly" stool?

7. What is the cause of the baby's eyes crossing?

8. Describe the anterior and posterior fontanels of a newborn. When are they expected to close? What is the significance of bulging when the baby is crying or sucking.

9. How significance is slight jaundice at 48 hours of age? Although this baby probably is experiencing physiologic jaundice, what other causes of jaundice must be considered?

10. Mother and Baby Taber are to be discharged this afternoon. Outline the teaching that the nurse should provide in regard to jaundice.

11. The mother states that she wishes to use breastfeeding for birth control. How should the nurse respond?

Questions and Suggested Answers

1. Baby Taber is the infant of a diabetic mother. What are the signs of hypoglycemia? Signs of hypoglycemia that Baby Taber might exhibit are jittery behavior and inability to maintain his temperature. **How is the baby tested for hypoglycemia?** The baby's heel is pricked, and a glucose reading is done on the blood. **What is the normal range blood sugar for a newborn right after birth?** A newborn's normal blood glucose is usually between 35 and 60.

2. Explain to the mother why the baby was given glucose water shortly after birth. Because the baby is used to getting high levels of sugar from the mother (diabetic) and has developed his own high insulin levels to deal with it, right after birth, when the glucose stops, the insulin will use up whatever glucose the baby has, causing a rapid development of low blood sugar. This can be dangerous. A small amount of 5% glucose or formula may be given to wean the baby off the high levels of glucose and allow him to gradually decrease his insulin production. A better alternative would have been to bring the baby back to the mother to breastfeed.

3. What other problems may occur in the infant of a diabetic mother (IDM)? These babies may also develop jaundice, respiratory problems, and low calcium and magnesium levels. Due to their large size and broad shoulders, these babies may experience birth injuries.

4. The mother distinctly told the staff that she only wanted the baby to get breast milk. The night nurse working in the nursery decided that, since the mother had had a cesarean section and had been nursing all day, she was tired, and that giving the baby one bottle of formula would give her a rest and would do no harm. Discuss this nursing decision and the validity of her conclusions. Although the nurse had good intentions of letting the mother sleep, this decision reflects poor nursing judgment. An infant that only receives breast milk also receives the maximal amount of protection from infection. Breast milk seals the infant's intestines and helps prevent the transport of harmful organisms into the baby's system. Giving the baby any other feeding, including formula, interferes with this process. Furthermore, for the mother to establish an adequate milk supply she needs to stimulate the breast on a regular basis. Missing a feeding interferes with her ability to produce an adequate milk supply and increases engorgement. Finally, offering a breastfed baby a bottle confuses some babies, making it more difficult for them to get back on the mother's nipple. The milk drips easily from the bottle and babies learn quickly the easy way to feed. Some will refuse to suck at the breast after getting a bottle. This is very discouraging for the mother. She feels rejected by her baby when the baby is looking for the easy way to feed.

5. Why is the baby now having problems latching on? There are two possible reasons for this.

- Nipple confusion, which occurs after a breastfed baby is given a rubber bottle nipple. The baby actually sucks differently from each.
- Engorged breasts make it difficult for the baby to latch on. Both of these could have been avoided if the nurse had taken the baby out to nurse at night rather than giving the baby a bottle of formula.

6. Discuss normal newborn stool patterns, including odor and consistency. Normally all babies will have dark meconium, which is black or green, sticky and tar-like without odor, for the first few days. By the second and third day the breastfed baby passes a transitional stool that is thinner in consistency and either greenish black or yellowish-brown and less sticky, and if totally breastfed will still remain odorless. By the fifth day a breastfed baby will then pass several stools a day that are thin and more liquid. These remain odorless unless the baby has received anything other than breast milk. It is not unusual for a breastfed baby at several weeks to go longer periods, up to one week to 10 days, without a stool. Breast milk is completely utilized by the baby, decreasing waste products. **What is the significance of a "smelly" stool?** This is an indication that bacteria have been established in the intestines as a result of the formula given the baby.

7. What is the cause of the baby's eyes crossing? Strabismus in the neonate is usually caused from muscle incoordination and gives the appearance of being cross-eyed. Pseudostrabismus, or the appearance of being crossed-eyed, may occur as a result of a flat nasal bridge, which is common in the newborn and also increases this appearance. This resolves by six months to one year.

8. Describe the anterior and posterior fontanels of a newborn. The anterior fontanel is diamond shaped and larger than the posterior fontanel, which is triangular. These are open spaces formed by the joining together of the neonatal head bones. **When are they expected to close?** The posterior fontanel closes first by two to three months and the anterior one usually is closed by 18 to 24 months. **What is the significance of bulging when the baby is crying or sucking?** If the fontanel bulges only when the baby is crying or sucking vigorously, this is normal.

9. How significant is slight jaundice at 48 hours of age? Since this mother is Hispanic, the yellow color may be a normal skin color. Blanching the skin and watching it return to its normal color can help eliminate this as a possibility. This is most probably from physiologic jaundice. It is caused by a normal increased breakdown of the RBC as the baby reduces his hematocrit to post-birth levels. It may also be a result of the mother having had an epidural anesthesia, having had Pitocin in labor, or from an excessive breakdown if the baby sustained bruises during the birth (unlikely with a cesarean section.) **Although this baby probably is experiencing physiologic jaundice, what other causes of jaundice must be considered?** Jaundice prior to 24 hours is always pathologic and requires immediate attention. Jaundice at any time may be a sign of infection, bile duct blockage, or inability of the liver to process the bilirubin as well as increased breakdown of RBC related to blood incompatibility. Additionally, infants of diabetic mothers experience increased jaundice levels related to breakdown of excessive RBC.

10. Mother and Baby Taber are to be discharged this afternoon. Outline the teaching that the nurse should provide in regard to jaundice. Babies that remain active, eat well and frequently, and pass several BMs a day are usually fine. Babies that become lethargic, are difficult to wake up, miss feedings, and just don't seem right need to be brought to the physician immediately. She should feed the baby frequently and not offer water or other supplements. She needs to take the baby undressed outside in indirect sunlight a few times a day and expose his skin to the sunlight. This will help reduce the jaundice.

11. The mother states that she wishes to use breastfeeding for birth control. How should the nurse respond? Many women in the world rely on breastfeeding for birth control. The method is called the Lactation Amenorrhea Method (LAM) and can only really be relied on for up to six months and then only if:

■ You totally breastfeed, including all night feedings (at least 6 feedings in 24 hours), and preferably do not use pacifiers.
■ You do not allow more than six hours between any feedings.
■ You have not had a period.

References

American Academy of Pediatrics. (2005). Revised breastfeeding recommendations. http://www.aap.org/advocacy/releases/Feb05breastfeeding.htm.

Blackburn, S. (2003). *Maternal, fetal, and neonatal physiology* (2nd ed.). St. Louis, MO: W. B. Saunders Co.

Littleton, L., & Engebretson, J. C. (2002). *Maternal, neonatal, and women's health nursing.* Clifton Park, NY: Thomson Delmar Learning.

Tappero, E., et al. (2003). *Physical assessment of the newborn* (3rd ed.). Petaluma, CA: NICU Ink.

Wheeler, L. (2002). *Nurse-midwifery handbook* (2nd ed.). Philadelphia: Lippincott, Williams & Wilkins.

Baby McMullen

AGE	**SPIRITUAL/RELIGIOUS**
24 hours	
SETTING	**PSYCHOSOCIAL**
▪ Newborn nursery	
CULTURAL CONSIDERATIONS	**LEGAL**
ETHNICITY	**ETHICAL**
▪ Hispanic American	
PRE-EXISTING CONDITION	**PRIORITIZATION**
CO-EXISTING CONDITION/CURRENT PROBLEM	**DELEGATION**
▪ Patent ductus arterosis (PDA); metabolic acidosis	
COMMUNICATIONS	**PHARMACOLOGIC**
	▪ Indomethacin (Indocin)
DISABILITY	**ALTERNATIVE THERAPY**
SOCIOECONOMIC STATUS	**SIGNIFICANT HISTORY**
	▪ Delivered by NSVD

NEWBORN

Level of difficulty: Difficult

Overview: The case requires that the student use critical thinking to assess a newborn with a murmur and identify the potential problems and best care for the baby.

DIFFICULT

Client Profile

Baby McMullen is a normal newborn delivered via NSVD after three hours of spontaneous rupture of membranes (SROM) at 36 weeks gestation. The labor, delivery, and pregnancy were without any problems. Her one minute APGAR was 8, and 9 at five minutes. She had an uneventful transitional period.

Case Study

She is now 24 hours old and has been doing well and feeding normally, but during an essentially normal routine examination she is found to have developed a mild grade I-II/VI SEM along the lower sternal border (LSB) radiating to the apex and axialia with an active precordium and full pulses.

Questions

1. What additional assessment should be completed for a newborn with a new onset murmur?

2. The nurse puts a call in to the physician. What laboratory studies should the nurse anticipate?

3. Which radiological studies should be anticipated?

4. The baby is feeding well, active, and has normal respirations and normal blood pressures. A patent ductus arteriosus (PDA) is diagnosed. Is the baby more likely to be cyanotic or acyanotic?

5. If the seemingly healthy baby's blood gasses came back demonstrating hypercarbia and metabolic acidosis, what would this indicate? Outline the support needed.

6. Should the nurse expect Baby McMullen's temperature to be unstable?

7. PDA may lead to pulmonary edema. Should the nurse anticipate strict I&O with fluid restriction and diuretics for Baby McMullen? Why or why not?

8. Would indomethacin (Indocin) be ordered? Why or why not?

9. List three risks associated with indomethacin, and indicate the special observations the nurse should be making while administering this medication.

10. If undetected and untreated, how might this baby's condition have progressed?

11. If Baby McMullen had been very premature, what additional problems might the baby develop as a result of the PDA?

Questions and Suggested Answers

1. What additional assessment should be completed for a newborn with a new onset murmur? The nurse should check the four extremity blood pressures to assess for a difference in systolic blood pressure. If there is a greater than 10-point difference when comparing right to left, and superior to inferior, the infant needs to be further assessed for a moderate- to high-grade coarctation of the aorta. This is a crude assessment of moderate- to high-grade coarctation of the aorta. While this is not very sensitive in picking up a coarctation, it is very specific in that no other aortic abnormality will give you this kind of finding when it is present.

2. The nurse puts a call in to the physician. What laboratory studies should the nurse anticipate? Initially, the pediatrician will probably order pulse-oximetry to assess arterial oxygenation present on room air. If this is abnormal, the baby's hemodynamics will be checked by getting right to left and superior to inferior readings. An additional test to be done, if the room air pulse oximeter is abnormal, is the hyperoxic test. This is done by obtaining an arterial blood gas from the left upper extremity after breathing 100% oxygen for at least 20 minutes. The normal results should be a PaO_2 greater than 200 mm Hg. If this is abnormal, an arterial blood gases (ABG) is then obtained from the right upper extremity in order to document any difference that might reflect the presence of a shunt. If any of these tests are positive, it would be reasonable to anticipate a CBC to assess for any early sepsis that may be present.

3. Which radiological studies should be anticipated? Image studies that might be indicated include an echocardiogram and chest x-ray (CXR). The echocardiogram is similar to the fetal ultrasound. It looks at the internal anatomy, flow, and some of the pressures. This is the definitive test to evaluate the status of the ductus arteriosus and the heart anatomy and to rule out other forms of congenital heart disease. The chest x-ray (CXR) is used to look for cardiomegaly by assessing the heart size. It may indicate signs of heart failure by showing the amount of fluid in the lungs. A large patent ductus arteriosus (PDA) will lead to pulmonary edema due to the increased flow through the lungs with diastolic volume overload; increased flow through the left atrium, left ventricle, and aorta; and left to right shunting to the pulmonary circulation (Blackburn, 2002).

4. The baby is feeding well, active, and has normal respirations and normal blood pressures. A patent ductus arteriosus (PDA) is diagnosed. Is the baby more likely to be cyanotic or acyanotic? This infant is not cyanotic because the blood flow would be from the oxygenated left across the ductus into the unoxygenated circulation of the lungs. If the baby was cynaotic, it would be an indication of a very complicated ductus that is only part of a larger and more complex picture of cyanotic congenital heart disease. In this case, the baby would also show obvious signs of distress such as poor feeding, lethargy, hypotension, cyanosis, tachypnea, and diaphoresis.

5. If the seemingly healthy baby's blood gasses came back demonstrating hypercarbia and metabolic acidosis, what would this indicate? Outline the support needed. The nurse should first consider lab error. This baby should demonstrate normal arterial blood gases (ABG) since the PDA in this case is asymptomatic except for the murmur. The test should be redone.

6. Should the nurse expect Baby McMullen's temperature to be unstable? Probably not. An unstable temperature is probably not related to the PDA. If Baby McMullen is unable to maintain her temperature, a separate problem may exist, possibly sepsis.

7. PDA may lead to pulmonary edema. Should the nurse anticipate strict I&O with fluid restriction and diuretics for Baby McMullen? Why or why not? Not for this baby. This is a near-term baby with an asymptomatic PDA. Strict I&O and use of diuretics would be required in a infant that was having trouble with right ventricular failure due to a large right to left shunting of blood from the systemic circulation over to the pulmonary circulation. These are usually very preterm babies. This shunting of blood places an overloaded strain on the right ventricle, causing pulmonary edema with obvious symptoms such as tachypnea, cyanosis, poor feeding, and lethargy. In these cases partial fluid restriction is used, but it is of limited use since the infant has a high need for fluid-based nutrition. If partial fluid restriction was not effective in controlled pulmonary edema, furosemide (Lasix) would be used to urgently control the congestive heart failure (CHF). It is important to note that furosemide must be used with caution since it alters prostaglandin metabolism and may, in itself, potentiate ductal opening.

8. Would indomethacin (Indocin) be ordered? Why or why not? Indomethacin is ordered in preterm babies with PDA because the preterm infant is sensitive to the prostaglandins and indomethacin is a prostaglandin inhibitor. Arachidonic acid metabolites (precursors to prostaglandin) keep the ductus open during the fetal period. Therefore, giving a prostaglandin inhibitor will aid in closing the ductus. This treatment would not be effective for this baby because she is so close to term that she has normal prostaglandin and has lost her sensitivity. What little effect Indocin would have would not be worth the toxicity of the drug.

In the preterm infant, the PDA is usually a result of respiratory distress syndrome (RDS), and the preterm infant is more responsive to prostaglandins. In this case the infant is nearly term, and the PDA is from either an opening that is too large, too closed, or associated with another condition such as persistent pulmonary hypertension of the newborn (PPHN) or ductal congenital heart disease. In these cases the underlying causes must be addressed.

9. List three risks associated with indomethacin, and indicate the special observations the nurse should be making while administering this medication. Complications with indomethacin administration to the neonate include:

- A transient decrease in the glomerular filtration rate and decrease in urine output. The nurse should keep very accurate I&O records.
- A slight transient bleeding in the GI tract. The nurse should check diapers for blood.
- Prolonged bleeding time and disruption of platelet function for 7 to 9 days. The nurse should be alert for signs of bleeding and easy bruising.

10. If undetected and untreated, how might this baby's condition have progressed? In this case the baby is nearly full-term, and the patent ductus arteriosus may simply be related to a normal delay in closure. This baby would probably have progressed without any serious events, and in a few days the ductus would have closed on its own. However, once a murmur is detected, it is important to rule out any of the more serious ductal dependent heart lesions that could become life threatening as the ductus closes and eliminates the necessary ductal shunt, which is keeping the infant alive.

11. If Baby McMullen had been very premature, what additional problems might the baby develop as a result of the PDA? In the very preterm infant, a PDA can be associated with prolonged ventilatory support with increased risk of bronchopulmonary dysplasia (BPD). Decreased perfusion of peripheral organ systems may occur due to inadequate systolic and diastolic flow. Decreased renal perfusion could result in the development of volume overload and congestive heart failure. Decreased gastrointestinal blood flow can result in intestinal ischemia and development of necrotizing enterocolitis (NEC). Cerebral ischemia may occur, resulting in intraventricular hemorrhage (IVH). Myocardial ischemia may also occur. Some of these infants require surgery to close the ductus prior to the development of any of these serious sequels.

References

Bianchi, D., Crombleholme, T., & D'Altom, M. (2000). *Fetology diagnosis and management of the fetal patient.* New York: McGraw Hill.

Blackburn, S. (2003). *Maternal, fetal, and neonatal physiology.* Philadelphia: W. B. Saunders Co.

Creasy, R. K., & Resnik, R. (1999). *Maternal fetal medicine* (4th ed.). Philadelphia: W. B. Saunders Co.

Taeusch, H. W. (2004). *Avery's diseases of the newborn* (8th ed.). Philadelphia: W. B. Saunders Co.

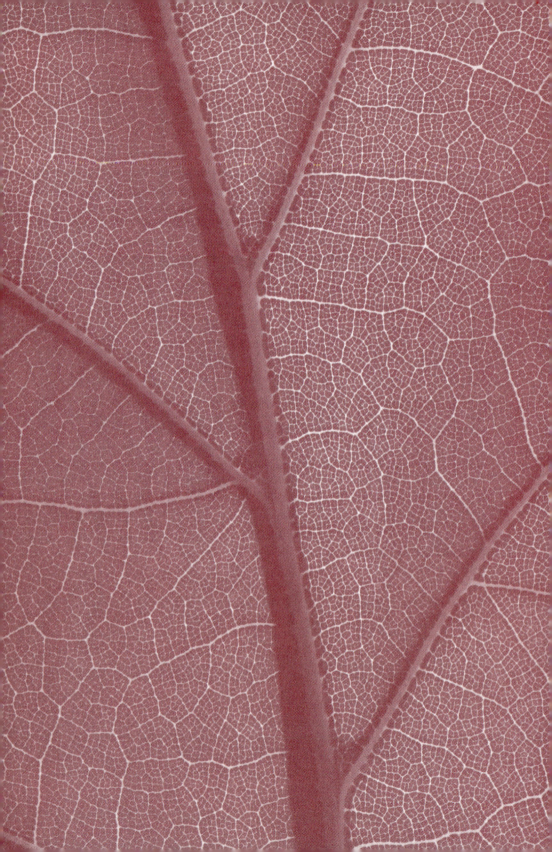

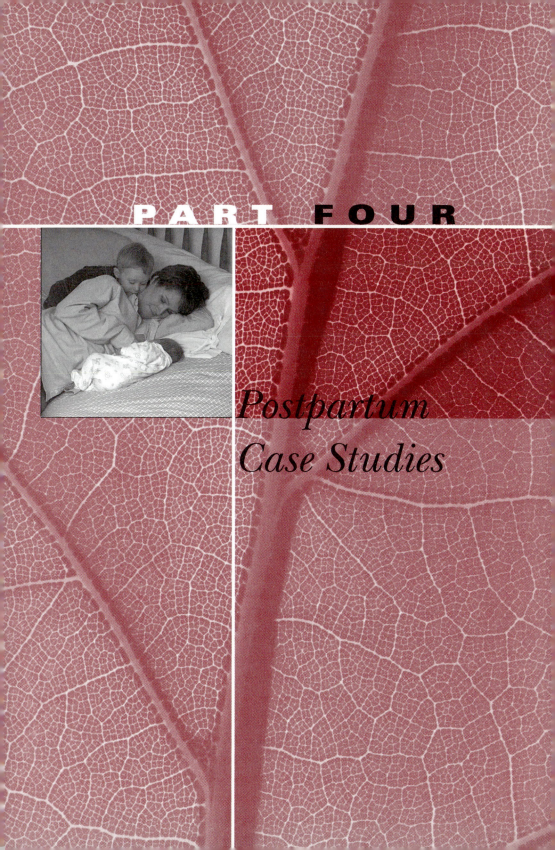

PART FOUR

Postpartum
Case Studies

CASE STUDY 1

Marie

AGE

38

SETTING

- Birth center

CULTURAL CONSIDERATIONS

ETHNICITY

- White American

PRE-EXISTING CONDITION

- Obesity; shoulder dystocia; postpartum hemorrhage; third-degree laceration

CO-EXISTING CONDITION/CURRENT PROBLEM

- Separated symphysis pubis

COMMUNICATIONS

DISABILITY

SOCIOECONOMIC STATUS

SPIRITUAL/RELIGIOUS

PSYCHOSOCIAL

- Previous positive home birth experience

LEGAL

ETHICAL

PRIORITIZATION

DELEGATION

PHARMACOLOGIC

ALTERNATIVE THERAPY

SIGNIFICANT HISTORY

- Multipara

POSTPARTUM

Level of difficulty: Easy

Overview: Requires using critical thinking to identify a separated symphysis pubis and provide care for the postpartum mother who is experiencing this complication.

Client Profile

Marie is a 38-year-old, G5P5005, MWF at two hours postpartum. She delivered her baby at the birth center. Marie is five feet one inch tall, and her weight at delivery was 160 pounds. Her delivery was complicated by a severe shoulder dystocia of seven minutes (Figure 4.1). The baby is doing very well after an initial resuscitation with positive pressure ventilation and oxygen. The 10-minute APGAR was 8, and the baby is currently nursing well. He is maintaining his temperature without difficulty and shows no further signs of respiratory distress. Marie's estimated blood loss was 700 mL following a third-degree laceration she sustained as a result of an extension of a midline episiotomy and the shoulder dystocia.

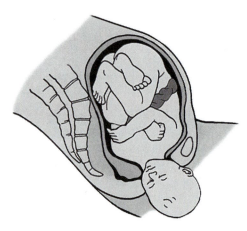

Figure 4.1 *Shoulder dystocia*

Case Study

At two hours postpartum Marie says she has to go to the bathroom. She is assisted to sit at the bedside for a few minutes prior to standing. When she does stand, there is a brief gush of blood from the vagina, and she cries out in pain. The nurse notes that there is swelling over the symphysis pubis, and the area is very tender. She also notes that when Marie stands, she does so with her feet pointing outward.

Questions

1. What is the most likely cause of her pain?

2. Why did the nurse have her sit at the bedside for a few minutes prior to taking her to the bathroom?

3. What explanation can be given for the brief gush of blood when she stood up?

4. What occurred during the delivery that could have contributed to the pain she feels when she attempts to stand postpartum?

5. Describe a third-degree laceration.

6. Assess her blood loss. Is it abnormal?

7. Will the mother need to be transported to the hospital immediately?

8. Outline the expected plan of care for Marie.

9. What is the prognosis for this condition?

10. Give two nursing diagnosis for this client.

Questions and Suggested Answers

1. What is the most likely cause of her pain? The most likely cause of her pain is a separated symphysis pubis. This occurs to a minor degree during many deliveries, goes undiagnosed, and has a spontaneous recovery. However, in rare cases due to traumatic labors associated with CPD and excessive abduction of the thighs at delivery, actual rupture of the pubic symphysis occurs.

2. Why did the nurse have her sit at the bedside for a few minutes prior to taking her to the bathroom? With the uterus now essentially empty, the abdominal organs can slide back into their original positions. This may cause some women to faint when they first stand after delivery. Sitting at the side of the bed for a few minutes before attempting to stand and walk may give her enough opportunity to adjust to the change and avoid fainting when she stands. The nurse should advise the new mother to call for help before she gets out of bed the first time after delivery. The nurse should also always have spirits of ammonia available in her hand when assisting a new mother out of bed for the first time following delivery.

3. What explanation can be given for the brief gush of blood when she stood up? When the mother is lying down, the normal lochia flow will pool in the vagina. When she stands, gravity will cause a slight gush from the vagina. The mother should be warned ahead of time and precautions made to catch the gush ahead of time. It should be noted that any time there is a gush of blood it should always be evaluated for possible hemorrhage.

4. What occurred during the delivery that could have contributed to the pain she feels when she attempts to stand postpartum? In this case, the mother experienced a severe shoulder dystocia. Her legs would have been placed in McRobert's position, severely flexed back and to the side. This position along with the efforts made to free the baby's shoulders are the most probable reasons for the separation of the symphysis pubis. Another contributing factor to this condition was very relaxed pelvic joints as a result of this being her fifth pregnancy.

5. Describe a third-degree laceration. A third-degree laceration extends through the perineal body, the transverse muscle, and the rectal sphincter. If not properly repaired the woman will be subject to fecal incontinence and high risk for ongoing infections.

6. Assess her blood loss. Is it abnormal? Average blood loss for a vaginal delivery is less than 500 mL. Her loss of 700 mL is excessive. Estimating blood loss can be difficult and is subjective. Compare predelivery and post-delivery hemoglobin and hematocrit levels to estimate the blood loss. Even in much higher blood losses there is not a significant change in hematocrit for 4 hours and it takes 48 hours for complete compensation to occur.

7. Will the mother need to be transported to the hospital immediately? No. Although this is very painful, it does not require an emergency transport. The mother will need to be evaluated for the degree of damage, and this may require an x-ray.

8. Outline the expected plan of care for Marie. Management consists of stabilizing the joint and pain relief. Depending on the degree of separation and the amount of pain, she may require several weeks of bed rest and a tight pelvic binder to stabilize the joint. A bed board under her mattress is recommended. The family should arrange for a trapeze to be installed over her bed to allow her to pull herself up without straining the pelvic joints. Obviously, she will need extra help at home to care for the baby and herself. A postpartum doula could supply this assistance. She will also need adequate analgesics. She should avoid stairs and use crutches as needed.

9. What is the prognosis for this condition? With adequate rest, the prognosis is very good. Only in rare cases is surgery needed.

10. Give two nursing diagnoses for this client. Nursing diagnoses appropriate for this client include:

1. Risk for thromboembolism related to prolonged bed rest postpartum
2. Alteration in parenting related to pain and inability to freely ambulate

References

Simpson, K. R., & Creehan, P. A. (2001). *AWHONN Perinatal Nursing* (2nd ed.). Philadelphia: Lippincott, Williams & Wilkins.

Wheeler, L. (2002). *Nurse-midwifery handbook* (2nd ed.). Philadelphia: Lippincott, Williams & Wilkins.

Cunningham, F. G., Gant, N., Leveno, K., Gilstrap, L., Hauth, J., & Wendstrom, K. (2001). *Williams Obstetrics* (21st ed.). London: Appleton & Lange.

Edith

AGE

36

SETTING

- Hospital postpartum unit

CULTURAL CONSIDERATIONS

- Mexican immigrant culture

ETHNICITY

- Hispanic American

PRE-EXISTING CONDITION

- Change in fob with losses accompanying second fob; previous spontaneous abortion; premature baby with congenital anomalies

CO-EXISTING CONDITION/CURRENT PROBLEM

- PP gestational diabetes; hypertension; blues; AMA

COMMUNICATIONS

DISABILITY

SOCIOECONOMIC STATUS

SPIRITUAL/RELIGIOUS

- Catholic

PSYCHOSOCIAL

LEGAL

ETHICAL

PRIORITIZATION

DELEGATION

PHARMACOLOGIC

- OTC Annusol, Preparation H; acetaminophen (Tylenol)

ALTERNATIVE THERAPY

- Nettle tea; grated raw potato; plantain and yarrow ointment; witch hazel

SIGNIFICANT HISTORY

- Grand multipara

MODERATE

POSTPARTUM

Level of difficulty: Moderate

Overview: Requires using critical thinking to assess postpartum changes and plan care for the woman with hemorrhoids. Requires assessing prenatal factors that increase pregnancy risks, including losses, advanced maternal age, and different fathers.

Client Profile

Edith is a 36-year-old, G9 P4326, Mexican immigrant, MHF who delivered a full-term baby boy weighing 9 pounds 2 ounces. She had a normal spontaneous vaginal delivery (NSVD) with no episiotomy or tears. She experienced a long prodromal early labor of over 10 hours. She refused Pitocin augmentation. Once she entered active labor, her labor progressed rapidly, and she was in active labor for six hours with a 30-minute second stage. The placenta was delivered spontaneously within 20 minutes. Her uterus has remained contracted. Her lochia is rubra moderate. Significant in her history is the fact that she had two spontaneous abortions and lost one baby due to prematurity with congenital anomalies. All of these losses have been in the past four years with her current husband. Her other children were with her first husband; all of them were born over 14 years ago and were completely normal. This pregnancy was complicated with hypertension (140s/90s) and gestational diabetes controlled by diet and exercise. She is five feet three inches tall, and her post-delivery weight is 186 pounds (8 pounds less than her last pregnancy weight done at 38 wga).

Case Study

Edith is now 18 hours post-delivery. Her main concerns at this time are severe afterpains and hemorrhoids. She is breastfeeding and the infant is alert, active, and nursing well, approximately every one and a half to two hours. During the night, the baby slept for four straight hours. Upon doing her assessment on Edith the nurse notices the following: BP 128/80; temperature is 99.4°, pulse 70, respirations 20. Her uterus is well contracted, midline, and the fundus is 3 cm below her umbilicus. Her lochia is rubra and she complains of afterpains. Her breasts are slightly engorged with the nipples erect without redness, she is voiding large quantities with each void without discomfort or burning, her perineum is slightly swollen, and she has not had a BM. She has one external hemorrhoid approximately 2 cm; several smaller external hemorrhoids also present and her Homan's sign is negative. The baby is nursing well with good latch on and positioning. The client is slightly teary and sad.

Questions

1. Give two possible explanations why this pregnancy was complicated by hypertension and gestational diabetes and her other previous pregnancies were not.

2. Assess Edith's vital signs. Are they normal?

3. Assess each of the nurse's observations.

4. Is there any significance to the fact that the earlier pregnancies were by a different father and the later ones, including the losses, were by a new father?

5. What nursing actions can provide relief for Edith's hemorrhoids?

6. Why are Edith's afterpains so strong?

7. What measures can be taken to give her relief?

8. How should the nurse approach Edith's emotional state at this time?

9. Assess the baby's nursing demand schedule. Is this normal?

10. Make a list of teaching priorities for Edith prior to her discharge.

Questions and Suggested Answers

1. Give two possible explanations why this pregnancy was complicated by hypertension and gestational diabetes and her other previous pregnancies were not. The hypertension may be a result of a reaction to the father's sperm. Hypertension in pregnancy is most often associated with first pregnancies and in grand multiparas. This includes first pregnancies with a new partner. The theory is that the father's sperm may result in a maternal reaction that leads to hypertension in the mother. Edith is a grand multipara, and her more advanced age and obesity with these pregnancies may contribute to hypertension. Gestational diabetes may be the result of her weight and advanced age. The fact that she is Mexican may increase her risk for pregestational diabetes, but not gestational diabetes.

2. Assess Edith's vital signs. A temperature elevation under 100.4° within 24 hours of the birth is usually a sign of dehydration, and she shows no other signs of infection. She is nursing frequently and should be encouraged to drink more. Postpartum pulses are usually low and hers is. Her respirations are fine, and her BP appears to be returning to normal. **Are they normal?** Yes. They are normal.

3. Assess each of the nurse's observations.

■ Uterus well contracted, midline, and fundus is 3 cm below her umbilicus and her lochia is rubra moderate; c/o afterpains.

Assessment: This is normal for this time PP. The fact that her fundus is already 3 cm below the umbilicus indicates good involution. The strong afterpains are a result of the multiparity and breastfeeding and are the reason why her involution is progressing so well.

■ Breasts slightly engorged, nipples erect without redness

Assessment: Engorgement is related to an accumulation of fluid in the breasts. Frequent nursing and allowing the baby to empty the first breast first may reduce this problem. Engorgement usually occurs around the third to fifth day. When the breasts are filled with milk, as when the baby misses feedings, the blood and lymph flowing through the breast slows and the fluid content of the blood enters the tissues of the breast, causing the engorgement. Engorgement may make it difficult for the baby to latch on, cause pain to the mother, and even account for a low-grade maternal fever (La Leche League, 2003). This finding is a little early; however, the baby was nursing every two hours, and has just slept for four straight hours, so this is normal. The major concern is to limit the engorgement and nipple trauma by encouraging the baby to latch on correctly and nurse frequently. Placing warm towels on her breasts prior to the next feeding may help.

■ Voiding large quantities each void without discomfort or burning

Assessment: This is normal; a diuresis occurs postpartum as the body readjusts its level of fluid after pregnancy.

■ Perineum slightly swollen; no BM; one external hemorrhoid approximately 2 cm; several smaller external hemorrhoids also present

Assessment: Slight perineal swelling is normal; hemorrhoids are not normal but a common finding. A bowel movement would not be expected at this early time.

■ Homan's sign negative

Assessment: This is normal; a positive Homan's sign may be an indication of a deep vein thrombosis (DVT). In addition to checking for Homan's sign, to assess for DVT the nurse also needs to be alert for signs of pain, redness, and warmth in the lower extremities.

■ Baby nursing well with good latch on and positioning

Assessment: This is normal. Breastfed babies drink more frequently than formula-fed babies due to the fact that they completely digest the colostrums/milk at each feeding and receive smaller amounts and therefore get hungry sooner. Latch on and position are very important since improper latching on and positioning are the most common causes of sore nipples.

■ Client is slightly teary and sad

Assessment: This is probably postpartum blues along with soreness from the hemorrhoids (which can be very painful) and afterpains.

4. Is there any significance to the fact that the earlier pregnancies were by a different father and the later ones, including the losses, were by a new father? The mother may be having reactions to the new father's sperm. The new father's sperm may also be defective since one baby was lost to congenital anomalies and prematurity and two were lost to spontaneous abortion. This baby needs to be carefully evaluated for any congenital anomalies, which may not be obvious immediately at birth. Her development of hypertension may also be associated with a response to this father's sperm.

5. What nursing actions can provide relief for Edith's hemorrhoids? The mother may find that sitz baths, cold compresses, witch hazel compresses (Tucks), local anesthetic spray, or local application of over-the-counter hemorrhoidal remedies such as Preparation H or Annusol can all offer relief from hemorrhoids. The mother, who prefers to use natural remedies, may wish to try one of several that have been reported to reduce hemorrhoids. These are nettle tea, one cup a day; locally applied grated raw potato to ease swelling and pain; and plantain and yarrow ointment to help relieve pain and shrink the hemorrhoids. Vitamin E supplements up to 600 international units per day may be helpful. The mother can be taught to lubricate her finger and push the hemorrhoid back inside the anus while lying down. It will remain inside while she is reclining and this will relieve both the pain and itching. Most often, hemorrhoids will reduce themselves over a period of 2 to 4 weeks postpartum. However, occasionally they will have to be surgically corrected if this does not occur. She needs to avoid constipation since straining will make the hemorrhoids worse. The physician/midwife will order stool softeners. These should be taken along with adequate fluids until the hemorrhoids are no longer a problem.

6. Why are Edith's afterpains so strong? Both the fact that she is a multipara and that she is breastfeeding will increase her afterpains.

7. What measures can be taken to give her relief? Keeping her bladder empty will help. (During early postpartum, the woman will often have reduced sensations of the need to void and have to be reminded to do so.) A mild analgesic such as acetaminophen (Tylenol) can be given just prior to nursing. Lying in the prone position will often reduce the cramping.

8. How should the nurse approach Edith's emotional state at this time? The nurse should accept that this is a common response to birth; he should use open-ended statements and avoid false reassurance. The most important thing is to provide time to listen to the mother. Let her go over her birth story and work through the experience. Give her the opportunity to resolve her problems as she sees them at this time or just to express her feelings. Postpartum blues usually resolves when the new mother can eat a regular meal and get a good rest.

9. Assess the baby's nursing demand schedule. Is this normal? Yes. This is normal. Nursing infants will often nurse for 20 minutes or so, sleep a short period (as little as 20 minutes), and then return to the breast for another short feeding. They may repeat this pattern several times during a feeding. This is normal and suits the normal digestive pattern for breast milk. Mothers need to be taught that they have adequate milk and not to provide supplements or pacifiers at this time. The return to the breast, providing increased stimulation, is what prompts the breast to produce additional milk.

10. Make a list of teaching priorities for Edith prior to her discharge. Edith is an experienced mother; however, it has been some time since she cared for a newborn. She needs a review of basic newborn safety and care and a review of her postpartum changes (lochia progression, her need for rest, and the danger signs (such as signs of UTI or thrombophlebitis). A referral to a La Leche League (LLL) group could prove very helpful for support during her nursing.

References

Biancuzzo, M. (2003). *Breastfeeding the newborn: Clinical strategies for nurses* (2nd ed.). St. Louis, MO: Mosby.

Blackburn, S. (2003). *Maternal, fetal, and neonatal physiology* (2nd ed.). St. Louis, MO: W. B. Saunders Co.

Gabbe, S., Niebyl, J., & Simpson, A. (2003). *Obstetrics normal & problem pregnancies.* New York: Churchill/Livingstone.

Littleton, L., & Engebretson, J. C. (2002). *Maternal, neonatal, and women's health nursing.* Clifton Park, NY: Thomson Delmar Learning.

Riordan, J., & Auerbach, K. (2005). *Breast feeding and human lactation* (3rd ed.). Sudbury, MA: Jones and Bartlett.

Weed, S. (1986). *The wise woman herbal childbearing year.* Woodstock, NY: Ash Tree Publishing.

Natasha

AGE

26

SETTING

- Hospital postpartum unit

CULTURAL CONSIDERATIONS

- Russian culture

ETHNICITY

- White American; Russian

PRE-EXISTING CONDITION

CO-EXISTING CONDITION/CURRENT PROBLEM

- PP depression

COMMUNICATIONS

DISABILITY

SOCIOECONOMIC STATUS

SPIRITUAL/RELIGIOUS

PSYCHOSOCIAL

- Isolation

LEGAL

ETHICAL

PRIORITIZATION

DELEGATION

PHARMACOLOGIC

- Fluoxetine (Prozac); paroxetine (Paxil)

ALTERNATIVE THERAPY

SIGNIFICANT HISTORY

- Multipara; elective abortion

POSTPARTUM

Level of difficulty: Difficult

Overview: Requires understanding the Russian culture. Requires using critical thinking to assess the influences of cultural isolation on postpartum adjustment.

DIFFICULT

Client Profile

Natasha is a 26-year-old, G2P0011, SWF. She is in a steady monogamous relationship with a man who is 54 years old. She is five feet seven inches tall, and her PPW was 128 lbs. She gained 52 pounds with the pregnancy. Her partner, whom she calls her husband, is an executive for a large construction firm. They met in Afghanistan, where Natasha was volunteering with the International Red Cross at one of the smaller hospitals, and Henry was overseeing a reconstruction project. Besides Russian, they both speak English and French. A year ago Natasha had a termination of pregnancy (TOP) after getting pregnant with Henry's baby when they decided that the time wasn't right for them. After much negotiating on where they would live and start a family, they decided to settle in Atlanta, Georgia, USA. Natasha loves the large city and is studying to be able to take the RN board exam in Georgia. Natasha and Henry still have mixed feelings about the termination of pregnancy (TOP), and when she got pregnant this time they decided they did not want to go through another abortion. Although she does get lonely for her family in Russia, Natasha is a very independent person and has generally adjusted well to her new life. Henry is extremely busy in his career, often leaving her for weeks at a time. Natasha finds it difficult to make new friends in Georgia. She is outspoken and always to the point, something many of the wealthy Georgia women are not comfortable with, and they sometimes find her to be "abrupt."

Case Study

Natasha is four weeks postpartum. She delivered a 9-pound baby boy at 41 weeks gestation at a planned home birth. Henry needed some convincing, but in the end he was very happy with the care they both received and the birth. Natasha was happy that she was able to feel that she was in charge of her birth, and the birth went beautifully. The baby nursed immediately and has been nursing well since. The only problem Natasha had with breastfeeding was some minor nipple soreness on day three and engorgement on day four. Henry had to go out of town one week after the baby was born to oversee a new project in Iraq. He plans to be gone for a month. Natasha has tried to go back to her studies. She has a maid who comes in several times a week to clean the apartment. Natasha did not make her follow-up postpartum appointment and is not answering her phone. The nurse from the birth center where Natasha got her prenatal care decided to do a home visit.

When she arrived she rang the door bell several times, and if she had not heard the TV on inside she would have left. After about five minutes Natasha answered the door. Natasha was in a dirty sweatshirt (milk stains down the front from her breast leaking and some smudges of food on the front) and her hair looked as if it had not been combed for several days. She was not wearing makeup (unusual for her). The baby was crying, and when the nurse saw him he was in clothes that looked like he had not been changed for several days. There was milk crusted along his neck, and he had a terrible diaper rash. The diaper did not look like it had been changed in at least a day. The apartment was cluttered. Natasha just looked at the nurse, invited her in, and quietly said, "Oh, I thought you were the maid. I think she is due to come this afternoon. It is Wednesday, right?" The day is Tuesday.

Questions and Suggested Answers

1. Distinguish between postpartum blues and postpartum depression.

2. What prenatal and postpartum factors may have contributed to Natasha's postpartum condition?

3. If Natasha is put on psychotropic medications to help with the depression, can she still breastfeed?

4. What signs did the nurse have that alerted her that she needed to do a home visit?

5. During the first few days postpartum,

what advice would have been appropriate for the nipple soreness and engorgement?

6. Outline what the nurse needs to do at this visit.

7. What professional referrals are needed?

8. What community resources can the nurse give Natasha?

9. What suggestions can the nurse give her at this time?

10. Is the baby at risk?

Questions and Suggested Answers

1. Distinguish between postpartum blues and postpartum depression.
Postpartum blues is a common emotional letdown response many women experience after the birth. It quickly resolves without professional help. Usually rest and good nutrition are all that is needed. Postpartum depression, on the other hand, is a serious complication that is often preceded by depression prior to the birth and often prior to the pregnancy. Many women experiencing postpartum depression lose track of reality. Inability to sleep or constant sleeping may occur. They feel a hopelessness that will not go away. Nutrition and sleep do not improve the condition. They may harm themselves and/or their baby and even other children. Not taking care of themselves and/or their baby, including even basic hygiene, are serious warning signs. They may isolate themselves. Professional therapy and often medications are needed. Thyroid imbalance may play a role in this type of depression.

2. What prenatal and postpartum factors may have contributed to Natasha's postpartum condition?

- She is far from home (Russia) and her family support
- Unresolved feelings about her TOP
- Her main support person is not with her
- She is in a different culture and is having problems making friends

3. If Natasha is put on psychotropic medications to help with the depression, can she still breastfeed? This would depend on the drug. Fluoxetine (Prozac) has been found to build up in the baby, but paroxetine (Paxil) does not. One recommendation is to avoid breastfeeding for 4 to 7 hours after taking any psychotropic drugs. If the baby is not breastfeeding at night, she may take medication just after the last evening feeding (Wheeler, 2002).

4. What signs did the nurse have that alerted her that she needed to do a home visit? Natasha missed her postpartum checkup and was not answering her phone. The nursing and midwifery staff that care for women who have home births follow these women closely. This is a holistic model of care, and it would be expected that a mother who did not return for postpartum care or answer her phone would be followed up with a home visit.

5. During the first few days postpartum, what advice would have been appropriate for the nipple soreness and engorgement? Observe her feeding and, if needed, suggest better ways to establish latch on and position to avoid trauma to the nipples. Engorgement is a transient condition that will usually resolve itself with consistent frequent breastfeedings. Warm towels and gentle breast massage (in the shower) will often provide relief. Cabbage leaves kept in the refrigerator can be put into the bra to help relieve the engorgement.

6. Outline what the nurse needs to do at this visit.

- Assess and change the baby.
- Assure the baby is not dehydrated and is nourished.
- Change the diaper and treat the diaper rash.
- Encourage Natasha to take a shower and change her clothes.
- Provide Natasha with nourishment.
- Discuss the need for having someone come to stay with Natasha all the time until her husband returns (a postpartum doula or live-in nanny may be helpful).
- Make an appointment for today with a mental health counselor or physician who specializes in postpartum depression. Make sure that she will go (arrange transportation, baby sitter, etc.).

- Have Natasha call her husband and explain the situation to see if he can cut his trip short or have a member of Natasha's family brought over to stay with her.
- If after assessing the situation the nurse feels it is safe to leave Natasha with the baby at this time, arrange to return the next day.

7. What professional referrals are needed? A mental health counselor or a clinician who specializes in postpartum depression can help Natasha.

8. What community resources can the nurse give Natasha? La Leche League (LLL) may be a source of social contacts for her, or there may be a new mother's group from the birth center she can attend.

9. What suggestions can the nurse give her at this time? Encourage her to talk. Explain that she is not the only woman to have ever gone through this, and with help she can get through it. Emphasize that she does need help; this is not just postpartum blues.

10. Is the baby at risk? The baby may be at risk. The baby is not only at physical risk from neglect, but women suffering from postpartum depression may injure or kill their babies. Even if no physical abuse or neglect were to occur, babies of depressed mothers are at a higher risk of emotional neglect. The baby's pediatrician should be made aware of the situation so that the baby's development can be carefully monitored. Women who are depressed may not talk to their babies or interact with them. This isolation is detrimental to the baby's development.

References

Baker, J. (2002, October). Treating postpartum depression. *Physician Assistant, 26*(10).

Biancuzzo, M. (2003). *Breastfeeding the newborn: Clinical strategies for nurses* (2nd ed.). St. Louis, MO: Mosby.

Riordan, J., & Auerbach, K. (2005). *Breast feeding and human lactation* (3rd ed.). Sudbury, MA: Jones and Bartlett.

Simpson, K. R., & Creehan, P. A. (2001). *AWHONN perinatal nursing* (2nd ed.). Philadelphia: Lippincott, Williams & Wilkins.

Wheeler, L. (2002). *Nurse-midwifery handbook* (2nd ed.). Philadelphia: Lippincott, Williams & Wilkins.

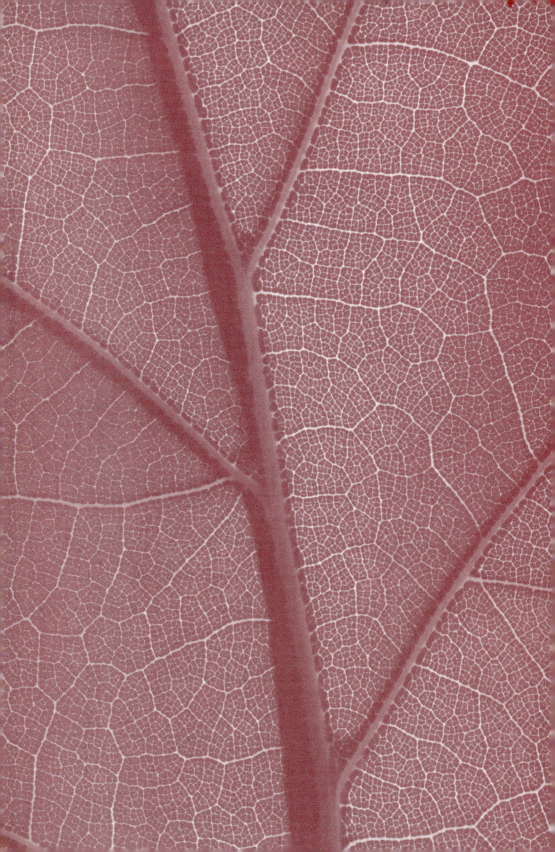

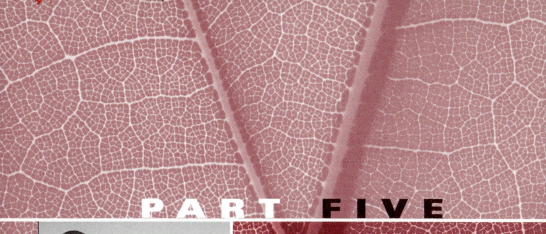

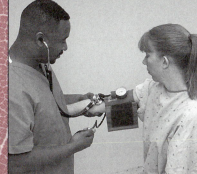

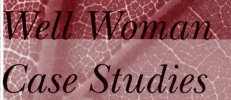

PART FIVE

Well Woman

Case Studies

JoAn

AGE

34

SETTING

■ Family planning clinic

CULTURAL CONSIDERATIONS

ETHNICITY

■ White American

PRE-EXISTING CONDITION

CO-EXISTING CONDITION/CURRENT PROBLEM

■ Late for Depo injection

COMMUNICATIONS

DISABILITY

SOCIOECONOMIC STATUS

SPIRITUAL/RELIGIOUS

PSYCHOSOCIAL

LEGAL

ETHICAL

PRIORITIZATION

DELEGATION

PHARMACOLOGIC

■ Depo-Provera

ALTERNATIVE THERAPY

SIGNIFICANT HISTORY

■ Multipara

WELL WOMAN

Level of difficulty: Easy

Overview: Requires using critical thinking to assess appropriate follow-up when a client presents at the clinic late for her Depo-Provera injection.

Client Profile

JoAn is a 34-year-old, G5P4105, MWF. Her last pregnancy was eight years ago. She has been using Depo-Provera for two years and is very satisfied with it.

Case Study

JoAn arrived at the family planning clinic this morning without an appointment. She appears upset and tells the nurse that she is late for her Depo-Provera shot because she had been at home sick with the flu for the past week.

Questions

1. How frequently should a woman repeat her Depo-Provera shots to be effective for contraception?

2. What questions should the nurse ask JoAn to determine if she should receive her next injection today?

3. List two common side effects associated with Depo-Provera injections.

4. What are possible signs of allergic reaction to the Depo-Provera injections?

5. JoAn's last injection was 14 weeks ago. Her urine pregnancy test is negative; however, she states that she had unprotected intercourse two days ago. What should the nurse advise?

6. JoAn states that, although she is not thrilled about another pregnancy, if she is pregnant she does not want to harm the baby and will carry it. List two other contraceptives that can be used to offer protection from pregnancy that can be used safely while waiting to see if she is pregnant.

7. How soon after intercourse can a pregnancy be detected?

8. What are the possible consequences to the fetus if JoAn is pregnant, did not know it, and got the Depo-Provera injection at this time?

9. List two long-term health effects associated with long term Depo-Provera use.

10. JoAn mentions to the nurse that she thinks her husband has not been faithful to her. How much STI protection does Depo-Provera provide?

11. List four mechanisms by which Depo-Provera prevents pregnancy.

Questions and Suggested Answers

1. How frequently should a woman repeat her Depo-Provera shots to be effective for contraception? Women are encouraged to have their Depo-Provera injections every 12 weeks. However, it is probably effective for at least 13 weeks.

2. What questions should the nurse ask JoAn to determine if she should receive her next injection today?

■ When was your last injection? *Note:* If records are available, they should be checked to validate her memory.

- Have you had unprotected intercourse since your last menstrual period?
- Has the unprotected intercourse been within the last 72 hours?
- Do you want to continue to use this form of birth control?

3. List two common side effects associated with Depo-Provera injections.
Common side effects with Depo-Provera are:

- Weight gain
- Spotting and bleeding
- Depression or PMS (although it may reduce these rather than increase them)
- Hypoestrogenism causing decreased libido, hot flashes, and increased risk for osteopenia
- Amenorrhea
- Severe headaches
- Acne
- Hirsutism

4. What are possible signs of allergic reaction to the Depo-Provera injections?

- Redness at the site may indicate allergy
- Anaphylaxis

5. JoAn's last injection was 14 weeks ago. Her urine pregnancy test is negative; however, she states that she had unprotected intercourse two days ago. What should the nurse advise?

- If JoAn does not want to carry a pregnancy and she had intercourse within the last 72 hours, she can be offered emergency contraception.
- Advise her to contact the office if she experiences signs or symptoms of pregnancy.
- Have her use a barrier method of birth control until her next period. If she has no menses for 14 days and then a negative pregnancy test, she may come in for another shot. She should use a backup method for another seven days.

6. JoAn states that, although she is not thrilled about another pregnancy, if she is pregnant she does not want to harm the baby and will carry it. List two other contraceptives that can be used to offer protection from pregnancy that can be used safely while waiting to see if she is pregnant.

- Condoms (male or female)
- Diaphragm or cervical cap

7. How soon after intercourse can a pregnancy be detected? A beta subunit human chorionic gonadotropin (hCG) test can detect pregnancy 7 to 10 days after conception.

8. What are the possible consequences to the fetus if JoAn is pregnant, did not know it, and got the Depo-Provera injection at this time? There are no known effects.

9. List two long-term health effects associated with long-term Depo-Provera use. Two of the more serious effects of long term use are:

- Potential for decrease in bone mineral density
- Rise in LDL and decrease in HDL

10. JoAn mentions to the nurse that she thinks her husband has not been faithful to her. How much STI protection does Depo-Provera provide? Depo-Provera injections do not provide any STI protection. Depo-Provera actually appears to increase a woman's risk of acquiring the sexually transmitted infections chlamydia and gonorrhea by approximately threefold when compared to women not using a hormonal contraceptive (NIH, 2004).

11. List four mechanisms by which Depo-Provera prevents pregnancy.

- Inhibits the LH surge, thus preventing ovulation
- Thickens cervical mucous, making it more difficult for sperm to enter into the female reproductive tract
- Causes slow tubal and endometrial mobility
- May alter endometrium to prevent implantation

References

Chan, P., & Winkle, P. (1999). *Current clinical strategies gynecology and obstetrics* (1999–2000 ed.). Laguna Hills, CA: Current Clinical Strategies Publishing.

Depo-Provera Appears to Increase Risk for Chlamydial and Gonococcal Infections. (2004). *NIH* (U.S. Department of Health and Human Services) *News* http://www.nih.gov/news/pr/aug2004/nichd-23.htm.

Hatcher, R. A., Nelson, A. L., & Zieman, M., et al. (2001). *A pocket guide to managing contraception 2001–2002.* Tiger, GA: Bridging the Gap Foundation.

Long, V., & McMullen, P. (2003). *Telephone triage for obstetrics and gynecology.* Philadelphia: Lippincott, Williams & Wilkins.

Lisa

AGE

32

SETTING

- Certified Nurse Midwife's office

CULTURAL CONSIDERATIONS

- Urban American White culture

ETHNICITY

- White American

PRE-EXISTING CONDITION

CO-EXISTING CONDITION/CURRENT PROBLEM

- Premenstrual syndrome; yeast infections

COMMUNICATIONS

DISABILITY

SOCIOECONOMIC STATUS

SPIRITUAL/RELIGIOUS

PSYCHOSOCIAL

LEGAL

ETHICAL

PRIORITIZATION

- Stress reduction; dietary changes

DELEGATION

PHARMACOLOGIC

ALTERNATIVE THERAPY

- Kava kava; St. John's wort; chamomile tea; valerian tea; melatonin

SIGNIFICANT HISTORY

- Multipara

MODERATE

WELL WOMAN

Level of difficulty: Moderate

Overview: Requires using critical thinking to identify timing of symptoms in relation to the menstrual cycle to assess for premenstrual syndrome and/or situational stress responses.

Client Profile

Lisa is a 32-year-old, G5P5005, MWF. Her youngest child is six years old and her oldest is 18. She is five feet three inches tall, and her current weight is 118 pounds. She has been working full time since her youngest child started school full time last year. She is a teacher's assistant. Lately there has been more stress at work since one of the other assistants went on maternity leave, leaving the school shorthanded. The additional work responsibilities have made it hard for her to get home from work at a regular time. Because of this she has had to ask her 13-year-old to be home for the youngest son right after school. He is resentful and has become increasingly moody. He has also started talking back to her and her husband. They are worried about the new friends he has made in junior high school. Her medical and surgical histories are benign; however, she has not had a physical exam since her last postpartum check up and lately she has been getting frequent colds. All of her children were born via NSVDs, and she breastfed the last three.

Case Study

Lisa is being seen in the well woman office today for a number of vague problems. Her husband insisted that she come in, stating that she is just not herself lately and something must be wrong. She is having problems sleeping at night and finds herself very short with everyone around her, especially her family. "Sometimes I hear myself just screaming, and I can't believe it's me. I am so ashamed of how I treat my husband and children at times, I just want to crawl in a hole and hide. I think they wish I would, too." Lisa has been relaxing at night lately with two or three mixed alcoholic drinks to help her sleep. This is not working. Her menstrual periods are normal for her and regular. She and her husband use condoms for birth control. She has been using an over-the-counter vaginal cream for repeated yeast infections, but it is not working very well.

Questions

1. List at least five questions that the nurse can ask Lisa to help identify the cause of Lisa's insomnia.

2. How effective is "a drink before bedtime" in helping a person sleep?

3. How does the stress in Lisa's life contribute to her current health problems?

4. What possible explanations can be given for the ineffectiveness of the over-the-counter medication for Lisa's yeast infections?

5. Give three possible causes for Lisa's mood swings and short temper.

6. What dietary suggestions can the nurse offer Lisa to relieve some of her symptoms?

7. How can Lisa fit an exercise routine into her busy schedule?

8. How might it benefit her?

9. How might Lisa's husband assist Lisa at this time?

10. Name at least three herbal and/or alternative therapies that might help Lisa.

Questions and Suggested Answers

1. List at least five questions that the nurse can ask Lisa to help identify the cause of Lisa's insomnia.

- Do you nap during the day?
- Do you always have trouble sleeping or only on certain days of the month?
- What time do you try to go to bed at night?
- How many caffeinated beverages (colas, coffee, chocolate, tea, etc.) do you drink, and when do you drink them?
- Do you exercise? If so, what kind, how much, and when?
- How late do you eat your last meal of the day?
- What do you do when you find you cannot fall asleep?
- Do you take any over-the-counter or prescription sleep aids?

2. How effective is "a drink before bedtime" in helping a person sleep? Alcohol may make a person feel sleepy; however, it can disrupt the brainstem sleep mechanism. This results in rebound insomnia.

3. How does the stress in Lisa's life contribute to her current health problems? Stress reduces the immune system's ability to fight infection. This probably accounts for her recent colds and yeast infections. Depending on her coping mechanisms and her ego strength, her immune response will be more or less affected. Helping her husband to understand her and encouraging him to support her will also improve her physical health.

4. What possible explanations can be given for the ineffectiveness of the over-the-counter medication for Lisa's yeast infections? She may have bacterial vaginosis (BV) or some other vaginal infection, not a yeast infection. The yeast medications available will not cure these.

5. Give three possible causes for Lisa's mood swings and short temper.

- Lack of sleep
- PMS (Premenstrual syndrome)
- Premature perimenopausal changes
- Life stressors

6. What dietary suggestions can the nurse offer Lisa to relieve some of her symptoms? PMS sufferers can benefit by reducing alcohol, caffeine, and refined sugar intake, and in increasing the fiber in their diet. Alcohol increases depression and interferes with sleep. Caffeine, even just one cup in the morning, can interfere with sleep. Refined sugar may contribute to depression.

7. How can Lisa fit an exercise routine into her busy schedule? She might try to get her son to take walks with her in the evening; this could give her some time alone with him. Thirteen-year-old boys often need more of their mothers' attention and do not know how to ask for it. This could address several of her problems.

8. How might it benefit her? Exercise is a wonderful tension tamer. Exercise releases beta-endorphins and lowers catecholamines. Both of these changes decrease depression. Exercise will also help prevent future health problems such as heart disease and osteoporosis.

9. How might Lisa's husband assist Lisa at this time? He might want to walk with her, offer a nightly massage to help her sleep, and try to help more with the children since she has just recently returned to the full-time schedule. Sometimes being patient and listening to her is all that is needed.

10. Name at least three herbal and/or alternative therapies that might help Lisa.

■ If Lisa's depression is mild and she is not taking a prescription antidepressant, she may try St. John's wort 900 mg divided into three doses a day. This will take several days before its effects are felt. If she is also anxious, she may try valerian 100–300 mg/day with the St. John's wort. Other helpful supplements are vitamin B_6 (50–500 mg/day) and vitamin C (1000 mg/day).

■ Chamomile tea, valerian tea, or melatonin are helpful to promote a natural sleep without hangover effects. Prescription sleep aids and even some over-the-counter sleep aids may be habit forming. They lose their effectiveness over time and require more to work. Sominex or Benadryl, sometimes used to promote sleep, can interfere with the production of the brain chemical acetylcholine, which is important for memory. According to Christiane Northrup, if these are used over a period of time they can cause serious memory problems and confusion (Northrup, 2001).

■ Occasional use of kava kava tea after very stressful days or when she feels anxious can help her sleep. Regular use should be avoided since it can be hard on the liver if taken in excessive quantities and may become habit forming.

■ Yoga, meditation, deep breathing, progressive relaxation, and imagery are all excellent ways to manage stress.

References

Libster, M. (2002). *Delmar's integrative herb guide for nurses.* Clifton Park, NY: Thomson Delmar Learning.

Northrup, C. (2001). *The wisdom of menopause.* NY: Bantam Books.

Sandy

AGE

38

SETTING

- Well woman clinic

CULTURAL CONSIDERATIONS

- Hispanic American culture

ETHNICITY

- Hispanic American

PRE-EXISTING CONDITION

- Eating disorder: bulimia
- History of gall bladder disease
- History of depression
- Family history of cancer and stroke

CO-EXISTING CONDITION/CURRENT PROBLEM

- Contraception; tobacco use

COMMUNICATIONS

DISABILITY

- Deaf

SOCIOECONOMIC STATUS

- Professional

SPIRITUAL/RELIGIOUS

PSYCHOSOCIAL

LEGAL

ETHICAL

- Client is considering single parenthood

PRIORITIZATION

DELEGATION

- Referral for exercise program

PHARMACOLOGIC

ALTERNATIVE THERAPY

SIGNIFICANT HISTORY

- Nulipara; history of gall bladder disease; history of depression; family history of cancer and stroke

WELL WOMAN

Level of difficulty: Difficult

Overview: Requires using critical thinking to assess the client risk and identify appropriate contraceptive choices for her.

Client Profile

Sandy is a 38-year-old, deaf G0, SHF. All through high school she was very afraid of gaining weight and kept her weight at 100 pounds or less. When stressed, she would vomit her food right after eating. Although she managed to control her bulimia during college and later during law school, she is still terribly afraid of getting fat. Sandy graduated from law school six years ago and is busy establishing her career. While in law school she had one severe gall bladder attack. It resolved on its own, but she is careful to avoid fatty foods. Just after her graduation she experienced a short period of severe depression. She was in therapy and on fluoxetine (Prozac) for about six months but is doing well now without it. She does not exercise. She would like children in the future but is not ready. At this time, she has not found someone whom she wishes to make a commitment to. Sandy smokes one pack of cigarettes a day. Her last check up was two and a half years ago. She does breast self-exams regularly. Her mother died of a breast cancer at age 42, and her father died of a stroke at age 49.

Case Study

Sandy has not used any birth control methods for the past two years, during which she had not been sexually active. She had used a combination birth control pill prior to that. Two months ago Sandy started dating two men and is considering becoming sexually active again with one or both of them. She would like a method of birth control that is easy to use and will not affect her ability to get pregnant if she should choose to do so. Sandy is five feet four inches tall, and her current weight is 119 pounds. She would like a method that does not have side effects. She is very afraid of gaining more weight.

Questions

1. While talking with the nurse Sandy mentions that she is afraid that "her clock is running out." She asks the nurse if using birth control will lessen her chances of having a baby in the future. What is the nurse's best response?

2. Sandy states that she is considering becoming a single parent. She asks the nurse what his opinion is of this option. The nurse's personal convictions are not congruent with deliberately bringing a child into a single-parent home. What are the ethical considerations that must be considered in this response?

3. Sandy has been deaf since birth. She asks the nurse what the possibility is that if she had a baby, the baby would also be deaf. What factors does the nurse need to consider in his response?

4. What should be included in her physical exam at this visit?

5. What specific risk factors need to be

considered when choosing a form of birth control?

6. Make a chart of available forms of birth control. Compare and contrast them for cost, ease of use, side effects, contraindications, effectiveness, and protection offered from STIs.

7. From the chart you made, choose two to offer Sandy.

8. Make a list of the teaching that the nurse would give Sandy for each of the two methods you chose.

9. Sandy's cholesterol level is checked and her LDL is 218 and her HDL is 37. Her triglycerides are 420. What is the significance of these findings?

10. Sandy states she would like to lose weight. Develop a diet plan for her.

11. She also tells the nurse that she wants to start on a serious exercise plan. The nurse asks the office receptionist to set up an exercise plan for Sandy. The nurse knows that the receptionist regularly attends a health club and uses a personal trainer. Is this delegation appropriate?

12. How does her history of gall bladder disease affect her choices for birth control?

13. What other health promotion advice can the nurse give Sandy?

Questions and Suggested Answers

1. While talking with the nurse Sandy mentions that she is afraid that her clock is running out. She asks the nurse if using birth control will lessen her chances of having a baby in the future. What is the nurse's best response? Generally speaking, delaying childbearing past 35 may increase chances of infertility regardless of the methods of birth control being used. Some forms delay fertility for a longer period of time than others. Also, complications that can occur during pregnancy are also greater after age 35. Older women are more at risk for hypertension and diabetes during pregnancy. Finally, after 35 the risk for having a baby with a congenital anomaly is greater.

2. Sandy states that she is considering becoming a single parent. She asks the nurse what his opinion is of this option. The nurse's personal convictions are not congruent with deliberately bringing a child into a single-parent home. What are the ethical considerations that must be considered in this response? The nurse must be careful in answering this question. If the client is asking for *personal* opinion, then the nurse may interject his personal beliefs, stating that they are his personal beliefs; however, if the client is asking about *professional* opinion, then the nurse needs to keep his personal opinion out of the response. If he is uncomfortable doing this, then he should refer her to a professional who can address concerns of single parenthood without personal bias.

3. Sandy has been deaf since birth. She asks the nurse what the possibility is that if she had a baby, the baby would also be deaf. What factors does

the nurse need to consider in his response? The nurse needs to know the cause of Sandy's deafness. Family history and her personal history will be important considerations. If Sandy had been exposed to teratogens prior to her birth, this may have caused her deafness and will not increase the risk for her children.

4. What should be included in her physical exam at this visit? Take a complete history and do a physical, including PAP and STI screen; CBC and blood glucose screen; offer a screening for the breast cancer gene; do a mammogram; and be sure she knows how to do breast self-exam (BSE) correctly. Her thyroid should be checked, and she needs a cholesterol screen done. She should be offered a baseline bone density screening because of her age and because she is a smoker, does not exercise, and had an eating disorder during adolescence during a time when she should have been building bone mass.

5. What specific risk factors need to be considered when choosing a form of birth control? She is at increased risk of STI because of new sexual partners. She has some high-risk factors for cardiac disease including high LDL, smoking, not exercising, a history of depression, a history of gall bladder disease, an eating disorder, and she may carry the breast cancer gene.

6. Make a chart of available forms of birth control. Compare and contrast them for cost, ease of use, side effects, contraindications, effectiveness, and protection offered from STIs.

7. From the chart you made, choose two to offer Sandy. The safest for her would be using condoms, either male or female. Sandy might be taught natural birth control. It would also have the advantage of making her more in tune with her body. This may help her later when she is trying to get pregnant. A cervical cap, or diaphragm, although it is not a popular method today in light of all the more convenient methods available, does offer the advantage of not increasing her other health risks. Because she smokes, is at risk for cardiac disease, is over 35, and has a family history of breast cancer, hormone methods are too risky.

8. Make a list of the teaching that the nurse would give Sandy for each of the two methods you chose. For the condom, review proper use. Discuss possible use of the female condom as an option. Natural family planning requires knowing how to identify the signs of fertility, documenting the observations, and being willing to abstain during the time of fertility. The cervical cap must be fitted; however, unlike the diaphragm, she will not have to be refitted if she gains or loses weight. She will need instructions on checking it for integrity, cleaning it, and knowing how long she can leave it in (to avoid toxic shock syndrome and cervical erosion).

Types of BC	OCP	Depo-Provera	IUD	Condom	Patch	Ring	Cervical cap	Dia-phragm
Cost	Yearly office visit	Q3 month Rx	One time/ requires Rx	OTC	One time/ req Rx	Req Rx	One time/ requires Rx	One time/ requires Rx
Effective-ness	99.6%	>99%	97–99%	96–60%	99%	98–99%	92–96%	97–80%
Ease of Use	Requires taking a pill at the same time each day	Requires injection q 3 months	Requires monthly checking for string	Requires use prior to every inter-course	Requires placement q month	Replace q 3 weeks	May be put in several hr prior to inter-course	Must be refitted if wt gain or loss of >10 lbs.
Side Effects	Depression; weight gain; menstrual irregu-larity; may contribute to osteo-porosis; HA; bloating; throm-boembolic disorders; acne; increased body hair growth; decreased libido	Weight gain; menstrual irregu-larity; may contribute to osteo-porosis; HA; bloating; depres-sion; thrombem-bolic disor-ders; acne; increased body hair growth; decreased libido	Irregular bleeding; cramping; May cause late spon-taneous abortion; potential for uterine penetra-tion	Allergy; decreased sensations	Allergy	Blood clots; heart attacks; stroke; hyperten-sion; risk of breast cancer; risk of gall-bladder disease; benign liver tumors; vaginal dis-charge; headache; nausea	Allergy; irritation of cervix	Allergy; increased UTI; TSS; may cause a foul smell
Contrain-dications	Pregnancy; throm-bosis; chest pain; severe hyperten-sion; known cancer; jaundice; diabetes w/compli-cations; unex-plained bleeding; age >35 and smoker	Thrombo-embolic disorders; breast or other reproduc-tive cancer	PID; dis-courage use with multiple sex part-ners	Allergy	Allergy	Pregnancy; throm-bosis; chest pain; severe hyperten-sion; known cancer; jaundice; diabetes w/compli-cations; unex-plained bleeding	Allergy	
STI Protection Offered	None	None	None	Yes	None	None	Some	Some

9. Sandy's cholesterol level is checked, her LDL is 218 and her HDL is 37. Her triglycerides are 420. What is the significance of these findings? Her levels are high and she is at risk for heart disease. Sandy has two risk factors for heart disease. She smokes and has a positive family history. Her total triglycerides should be under 200 mg/dL. Her LDL should be under 160 mg/dL. Her HDL, the good cholesterol, needs to be at least 40 mg/dL. Although these levels need correcting, she is premenopausal and her LDL is under 219 mg/dL; therefore, according to the American Heart Association, she is not a candidate for cholesterol-lowering drug therapy. She can reduce her risk for heart attack by limiting her intake of carbohydrates and including foods that increase HDL and reduce her triglycerides, such as products with monounsaturated and polyunsaturated fats, by starting an exercise program that includes at least 30 minutes every day, and by quitting smoking.

10. Sandy states she would like to lose weight. Develop a diet plan for her. This client is not overweight, but she has a history of eating disorders. Her concern over her weight may open an opportunity for the nurse to help her develop healthy eating habits. To improve her cardiac health she needs foods that are low in cholesterol, carbohydrates, and fat, in well-balanced and small portions. Eliminate all sodas and replace them with water. Eliminating sodas, especially colas and root beers, will reduce bone loss. She should be given a list of the omega-3 polyunsaturated fats to include in her diet as these play a role in lowering blood cholesterol. These are found in fish and fish oils. To further decrease her risk for osteoporosis, Sandy needs to increase her calcium intake and match it with magnesium (2:1). Trace minerals manganese, zinc, and copper have also been shown to be helpful in increasing the calcium absorption for prevention of osteoporosis.

11. She also tells the nurse that she wants to start on a serious exercise plan. The nurse asks the office receptionist to set up an exercise plan for Sandy. The nurse knows that the receptionist regularly attends a health club and uses a personal trainer. Is this delegation appropriate? No, this is not appropriate. The office receptionist is not qualified to advise Sandy. The nurse is aware of Sandy's overall health risk and needs. He needs to advise Sandy to exercise by starting slow, warming up, and cooling down afterwards, and to stop if chest pain develops. The nurse is aware of the need to include exercises that are weight bearing to reduce risk for osteoporosis. He should advise Sandy to establish a regular pattern and stay with it. She should exercise every day if possible for at least thirty minutes. This can increase her energy level, decrease her risk for osteoporosis, lower her cholesterol, and provide overall health improvement.

12. How does her history of gall bladder disease affect her choices for birth control? Women with gallbladder disease should avoid hormone based birth control as these methods may make the problems worse.

13. **What other health promotion advice can the nurse give Sandy?** She needs to stop smoking and use protection against STIs.

References

American Heart Association. (2005). What are healthy levels of cholesterol? Retrieved June 1, 2005, from http://www.americanheart.org/presenter.jhtml?identifier=183.

Morgan, G., & Hamilton, C. (2003). *Practice guidelines for obstetrics and gynecology* (2nd ed.). Philadelphia: Lippincott, Williams & Wilkins.

National Heart, Lung and Blood Institute. (2004). www.hhlbi.nih.gov.

Whitney, N., Cataldo, C. B., & Rolfer, S. R. (2002). *Understanding normal and clinical nutrition.* Belmont, CA: Thompson/Wadsworth Learning.

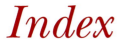

Index

Page numbers in **bold** indicate figures.

THOMSON

DELMAR LEARNING

™

Thomson Delmar Learning's Case Studies Series: Maternity and Women's Health
by Diann S. Gregory

Vice President, Health Care Business Unit:
William Brottmiller

Editorial Director:
Cathy L. Esperti

Executive Editor:
Matthew Kane

Developmental Editor:
Maria D'Angelico

Editorial Assistant:
Michelle Leavitt

Marketing Director:
Jennifer McAvey

Production Director:
Carolyn Miller

Production Editor:
Jack Pendleton

COPYRIGHT © 2006 by Thomson Delmar Learning. Thomson, the Star logo, and Delmar Learning are trademarks used herein under license.

Printed in Canada
1 2 3 4 5 XXX 10 09 08 07 06 05

For more information, contact Thomson Delmar Learning,
5 Maxwell Drive,
Clifton Park, NY 12065
Or find us on the World Wide Web at http://www.delmarlearning.com

ALL RIGHTS RESERVED. No part of this work covered by the copyright hereon may be reproduced or used in any form or by any means—graphic, electronic, or mechanical, including photocopying, recording, taping, Web distribution or information storage and retrieval systems—without the written permission of the publisher.
For permission to use material from this text or product, contact us by
Tel (800) 730-2214
Fax (800) 730-2215
www.thomsonrights.com

Library of Congress Cataloging-in-Publication Data

Gregory, Diann S.
  Maternity and women's health / Diann S. Gregory.
    p. ; cm.—(Thomson Delmar learning's case studies series)
  Includes bibliographical references and index.
  ISBN 1-4018-2711-X (pbk.)
  1. Maternity nursing—Case studies.
  2. Gynecologic nursing—Case studies.
  [DNLM: 1. Maternal-Child Nursing—Case Reports. 2. Women's Health—Case Reports. WY 157.3
  G822m 2006] I. Title. II. Series.
  RG951.G743 2006
  618.1′0231—dc22
                                    2005005765

Notice to the Reader

Publisher does not warrant or guarantee any of the products described herein or perform any independent analysis in connection with any of the product information contained herein. Publisher does not assume, and expressly disclaims, any obligation to obtain and include information other than that provided to it by the manufacturer.

The reader is expressly warned to consider and adopt all safety precautions that might be indicated by the activities described herein and to avoid all potential hazards. By following the instructions contained herein, the reader willingly assumes all risks in connection with such instructions.

The publisher makes no representations or warranties of any kind, including but not limited to, the warranties of fitness for particular purpose or merchantability, nor are any such representations implied with respect to the material set forth herein, and the publisher takes no responsibility with respect to such material. The publisher shall not be liable for any special, consequential, or exemplary damages resulting, in whole or part, from the reader's use of, or reliance upon, this material.

THOMSON DELMAR LEARNING'S
CASE STUDY SERIES

Maternity

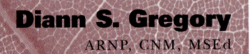

&

Women's Health

Diann S. Gregory
ARNP, CNM, MSEd

Professor of Nursing and Midwifery
Miami Dade College, Miami, Florida

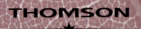

THOMSON
™
DELMAR LEARNING

Australia   Canada   Mexico   Singapore   Spain   United Kingdom   United States